ROGERS' SCHOOL OF HERBAL MEDICINE

VOLUME ELEVEN:

LYMPHATIC SYSTEM

ROBERT DALE ROGERS RH (AHG)

COVER
Top: Western Blue Flag
Middle: Common Figwort flowers
Bottom Left: Pokeweed berries
Bottom Right: Sweet Clover

This book is for educational purposes only. The suggestions, recipes and historical information are not meant to replace a medical advisor. The author assumes no liability for unwise or unsafe usage by readers of this book.

For those interested in using herbal medicine, seek the advice of a professional.

TABLE OF CONTENTS

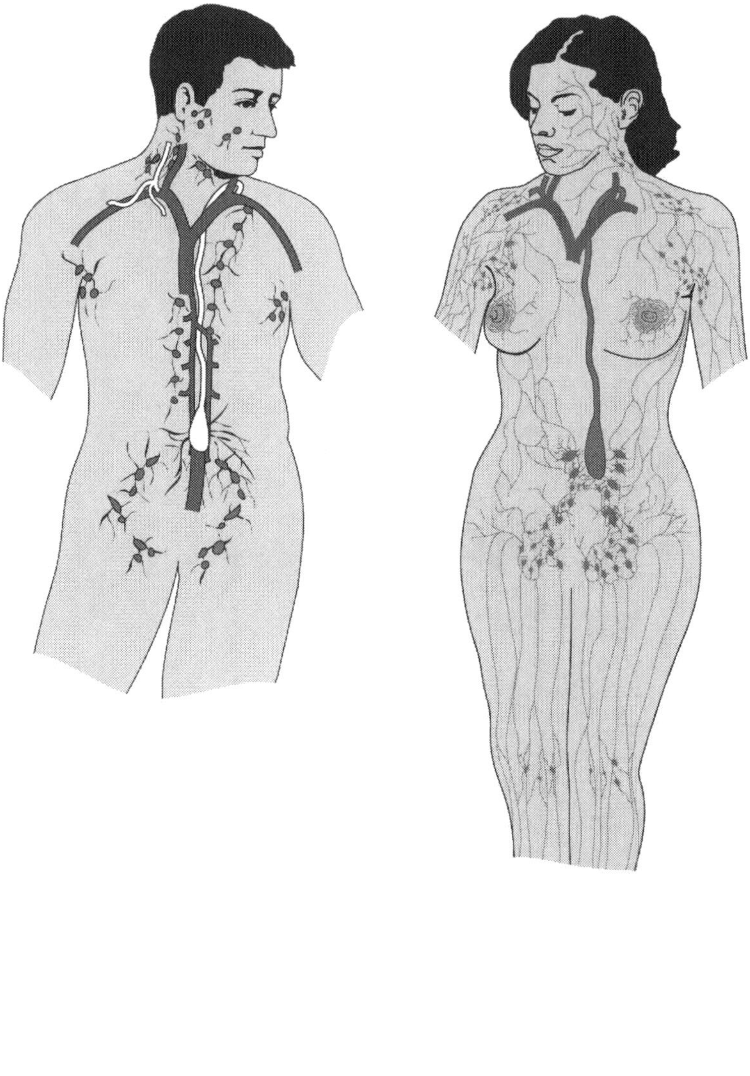

THE LYMPHATIC SYSTEM

The lymphatic system and immune system are integrated. I have separated the two for several reasons, but mainly to allow me to share more plants with you.

First let us look at the anatomy of this system.

In ancient Greece, congesting and swelling of lymphatic nodes was called scrofula.

The main nodes are found in the neck, under the arms, sides of breast and groin area.

Various parts of the lymphoid tissue are found in the spleen, thymus, Peyer's patches, appendix, tonsils and adenoids, and even the liver.

The lymphatic system has three times the volume of blood in the cardiovascular system, and yet is not "pumped". In and out movements of the diaphragm help move the interstitial fluid that bathes each and every cell of our body.

In turn, the fluid provides nutrients to the cells and of course moves waste out.

It has been found ten minutes on a trampoline is equivalent in benefit to the lymphatic system as a one hour jog!

Lymphatic drainage massage can be beneficial to those with chronically swollen nodes, or in cases of lymphoedema, especially if associated with breast surgery and removal of lymphatic nodes.

The cell walls have a positive charge so they repel each other and keep from sticking together.

Blood in the capillaries feeds the interstitial fluid and in turn the cells. Carbon dioxide, excess water, various salt compounds and small protein can move back into the veins, but larger protein, dead waste and bacteria need another route.

Lymphatic capillaries become tubes with nodes in which the lymph is filtered. In these glands are white blood cells that break protein into smaller chunks. These white blood cells are able to cross tissue membranes and go back into interstitial fluid. They move to the liver and kidneys for decision-making time; what to keep, recycle or throw out.

Rapid movement or quick lymphatic cleansing can cause discomfort and a form of auto-intoxication if the waste moves too quickly into the bloodstream.

Lymphatic tissue also drains the membranes of the small intestine via a lacteal. Blood vessels pick up sugars and protein of three amino acids or smaller, and the lacteals absorb fats and lipids and move them to larger lymphatic ducts for filtering.

Of course, it is all more complicated than this, and this is not a book on physiology but on herbs. Let's get started.

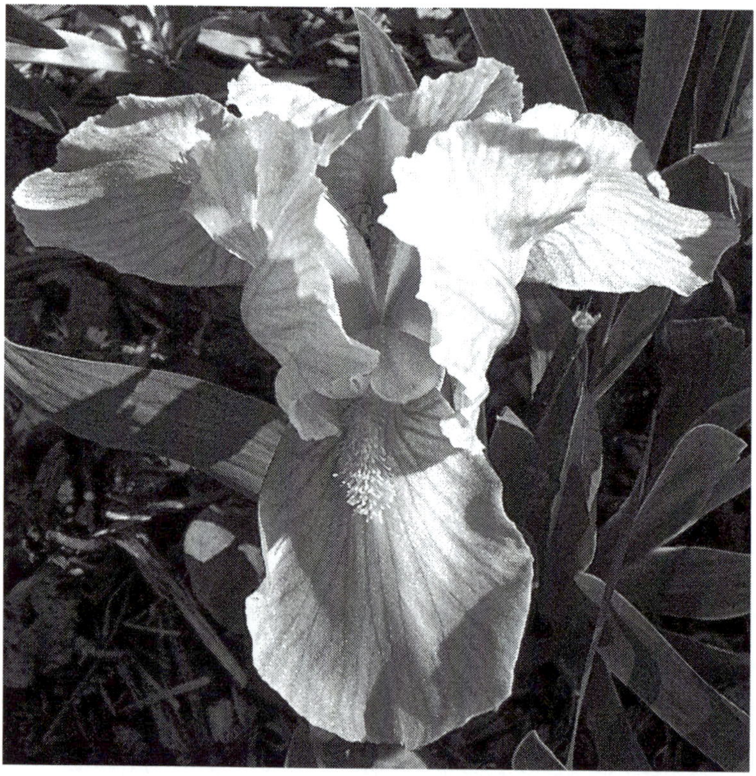

Iris

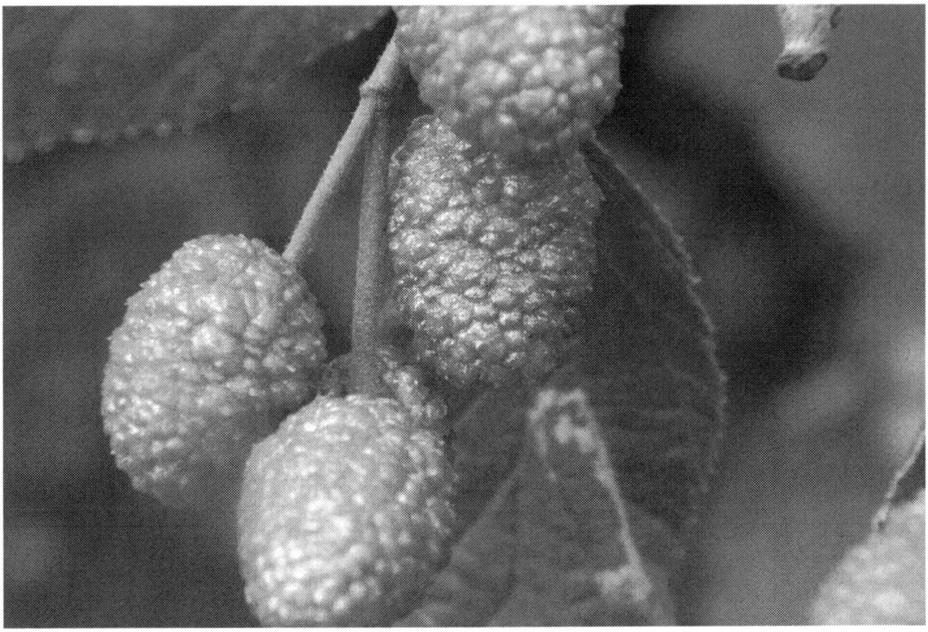

Green Alder cones

GREEN ALDER
(*Alnus crispa* [Ait.] Pursh**)**
(*A. viridis* ssp. *crispa* [Ait] Turrill**)**
(*A. viridis* [Vill.] Lam. & DC.)
(***A. viridis* ssp. *fruticosa***)
SITKA ALDER
(*A. sinuata*)
(*A. sitchensis*)
(*A. viridis* ssp. *sinuata* [Regel] Hult.**)**
RIVER ALDER
MOUNTAIN ALDER
THIN LEAF ALDER
(*A. incana* ssp. *tenuifolia* [Nutt.] Breitung**)**
(*A. tenuifolia* Nutt.**)**
SPECKLED ALDER
SMOOTH ALDER
GRAY ALDER
(*A. incana ssp. rugosa* [Du Roi] Clausen**)**
(*A. rugosa* [Du Roi] Spreng.**)**
PARTS USED- catkins, leaf, bark

The Alder, whose fat shadow nourisheth
Each plant set neere to him flourisheth. **WILLIAM BROWNE**

The meadows were veiled in a low creeping haze, through which tufts of Alders peered out like puffs of dark smoke. **POLISH SAYING**

I thought the sparrow's note from heaven
Singing at dawn in the alder bough.
I brought him home in his nest at even,
He signs the song, but it cheers not now,
For I did not bring home the river and sky. **EMERSON**

Alnus is from the Anglo Saxon **ALR**, the Old English **ALOR** and in turn from the Old German **ELAWER** or **ELO** meaning, "reddish-yellow". It progressed to **ALER**, then **ALLER**, or **ALDIR** to today's form.

The German term **ALUZA** may be from Indo-European **ALISA**. Alys was the name of the goddess of the burial island. It is possible the Elysian fields, or "islands of souls" were originally found in similar rivers.

The color is from the characteristic of wood to change color after felling. **INCANA** is from Latin meaning light gray, in reference to the white under leaf. **CRISPUS** meaning curled, and **TENUFOLIA** means, thin leaves.

At one time it was considered unlucky to fell an alder, most interesting considering that the city of Venice is built on alder and larch posts. The wood hardens like iron under water, and makes long lasting bridges, jetties, sluices and pumps.

The ancient Greeks considered alder sacred to Cronos, the God of Time. Its Greek name **KLETHRA** is derived from kleio meaning, "to surround or enclose". They were considered the transformed sister of Phaeton, the son of Helios and brother of Circe.

In Scotland, the wood was valued for construction and known as Scottish Mahogany, due in part to the rust colour of the new cut wood and sap.

The Alder represents the letter F (fearn) in the Druidic tree alphabet. It was known in medieval legend as the tree of the Erl King, sacred to the Celtic God Bran, the brother of Branwen, who kept the cauldron of Regeneration. His name means crow or raven.

Bran is a god of the dead, who carries a cauldron that brings the dead back to life. The cult of Bran was melded with the cult of Teutates, who drowned humans in alder groves. Later, both were transformed into the Fisher King to accommodate Christian myth.

This cauldron was the womb of the Great Goddess of paleolithic times, and thus is the fountain of youth.

In the famous *Battle of the Trees*, from a 10th century Welsh poem, followers of Bran wore alder sprigs. Fatally wounded, he had them cut off his head and carry it to a secret island (Avalon?) where for 80 years he told stories and sang songs. Other versions tell of his head remaining alive for 80 years on the way to London before being buried in the White Hill beneath the Tower of London. The purple of the buds is associated with Bran, and known as royal purple.

In the territory of Celtic Druids there was at one time a tribe known as Averni, or People of the Alder. In Irish legend, the first human male was created from alder, and the first female human from mountain ash.

In fact, one female figure, representing Alder Woman, carved from alder and dated between 728 and 524 BC, has been found in a peat bog on the west coast of Scotland. Across the sea, in Ireland, the wood was carved into wooden clogs for dry, warm footwear.

Alder is associated with the God Neptune, planet Venus, and the astrological signs of Cancer and Pisces (water).

In Norse legends, the month of March was associated with the waking Alder, and known as Lenet. This was a time of enforced fasting due to lack of food, and became the origin of the Christian festival of Lent. Alder is also associated with the 11th Norse Rune, IS.

Alder is our only broad-leaved tree to produce cones. These ripe, green cones were decocted in water in parts of England and drunk daily to alleviate gout.

The alder of Northern Alberta would be considered a tall, spreading shrub rather than a tree. The branches have a somewhat sticky surface that can be used as natural flypaper.

Alders are natural nitrogen fixers, like clover, and change atmospheric nitrogen into a form plants can use as fertilizer. They are valuable for restoring and regenerating mined and oil sand sites, checking erosion, and building up organic content.

These pioneer trees add the equivalent of ten bags of high nitrogen fertilizer to every hectare per year. It has been estimated that the leaves, when shed, provide another 160 kilos of nitrogen per hectare of soil. Inter-planting with hybrid poplar increases growth.

Green Alder is a very protein rich source of food that is virtually never browsed by moose or mice. This may be due to the presence of pinosylvan methyl ether, a strong herbivore repellant and abortifacient. In fact, this same compound extracted from tropical plants, is used as a wood preservative at low concentrations, protecting wood from termites for over two years.

Metal binding, histidine-rich proteins have been isolated from the root nodules of Alder, suggesting some potential in bioremediation. Gupta RK et al, *Journal Protein Chem* 2002 21:8.

Experiments in Holland have shown growing alders in an apple orchard raised fruit yield by 36%.

It is much prized for smoking fish or game due to the mild flavor and slow burning properties of the wood. When well dried it produces a hot fire that doesn't throw sparks and leaves little ash. It is not as rich in BTUs as birch, but much better than aspen or pine.

The Cree call it **ATOSPI** or **MISKWATOSPI** and use the plant in a variety of ways. The dormant bark was stripped and dried for dying hides used for clothing and moccasins. The bark was mixed with animal fats for body paint in traditional dances.

The Flathead boiled the bark for a bright red dye. They sometimes used this to produce odd-looking bright orange hair. Alder contributes a number of dye colors. The flowers give a green dye, the bark a fiery red, the young shoots cinnamon, and with copper mordant a pure yellow.

The Eastern Cree call Green Alder, **NEPATIHE**, and used bark decoctions to treat dropsy.

Speckled Alder is known, to Potawatomi as **ATOB**, meaning bitter. The inner bark was used for itchy skin and a bark tea for vaginal infections and as enema for hemorrhoids.

The wood can be carved into pipes, form the framework of birch bark baskets, or bent into small bows for hunting squirrels or birds.

A pipe stem can be made by sealing a grub into one end of an alder stem, forcing the insect to burrow its way out the other end.

The natural curve commonly found at the base of the shrub can be carved and fire hardened to peel bark from other trees. The wood was traditionally used to make the bottom and lid of birch bark containers, including one for beaver castors.

Work at the University of Maine in the 1960s, showed alder makes good kraft pulp, or can be chipped for hardwood composite board.

The rotten wood makes a good smudge, a smoke for tanning hides, or smoking fish. This dry rot was traditionally mixed with powdered willow bark for burns, in the form of a poultice.

Alder walking sticks, made from rotting branches, were lit and smoldered as a traveling mosquito repellant. The drifting smoke kept them away, and the periodic waving of the stick kept the fire slowly smoldering.

The fresh leaves were crushed and used as a poultice by nursing mothers with sore or swollen breasts. If the fresh leaves are ground and combined with small amount of warm milk, a suitable cheesecloth poultice can be used. The crushed leaves will relieve pain and decoctions of the leaves will quickly relieve sore feet when soaked in a warm footbath.

Leaves, with the morning dew still clinging, are placed in areas of the home having problems with fleas. They are attracted to the resins and can then be gathered and removed.

Various western tribes injected cool alder enemas to soothe bleeding hemorrhoids.

The Blackfoot used hot bark decoctions internally to heal tuberculosis of lymph glands in the neck. They call it **A-MUCK-KO-IYSTIS**, or red mouth bush, caused by chewing the bark.

The Dene people used the dried green cones, finely chopped, in smoking mixtures.

Both Dene and Cree of northern Saskatchewan boiled the green female catkins to treat venereal disease in men. The stems were boiled as an emetic for upset stomach.

The roots are dug up and decocted to relieve menstrual cramps or used as part of a steam/sweat to bring on menstruation.

The Chipewyan of northern Alberta know green alder as **K'AI LISEN**, or "willow that smells".

Further north on the Mackenzie delta, the Gwich'in call the plant red willow, or **K'OH**. Sophie Thomas, a Sai'Kuz healer, used bark shavings of **K'US** for cancers and ulcers, and sores in baby's mouth. It was combined with raspberry and chokecherry as a wash for skin ulcer and cancers including leukemia.

They used the inner bark to dye hides, skins, snowshoe frames and fish nets. Animal hides, for example, were soaked in a cool bark solution for 24 hours.

The inner bark was pounded and rolled up in beaver and wolverine skins to make them softer. This same decoction was used to revive worn moccasins, or at least restore and re-condition them.

For various human skin conditions, the bark was peeled from the stem, boiled, and cooled. The liquid, including the oily film on surface, was bathed on skin sores, scabs, eczema, sunburn and rashes. Stiff, arthritic joints were likewise treated.

The small green cones were chewed and the juice swallowed to relieve colds.

The Dena'ina of Alaska call this species fire willow or **QENQ'EYA**. It is used for fish traps and net-like drags, and digging sticks. The inner bark is boiled and taken for gas and to relieve fever. Like others, the bark was used to dye skin, and wooden objects, the latter preserved by rubbing animal fat over the newly dyed wood.

Alder roots can be split and used as twine if spruce or tamarack roots are not available.

The Nlaka'pamux used the fragrant stems of mountain alder as a perfume, and the small twigs for basket ornamentation. The Okanagan people made a string from the bark of young alder, as well as coiled baskets from the peeled, split and soaked roots.

The Gitksan name is **AMLUUX**, meaning neck ring, in reference to a special neck ring worn by chiefs and shamans composed of red cedar inner bark dyed red from alder bark decoctions.

Thin-leaf Alder (*A. incana*) was used by the Dena'ina for a similar purpose. Some say it should not be used for cooking as the red juice looks like blood when it is burning. The red juice from tea is taken to treat tuberculosis.

This same dye was used for woven maple baskets and wool. After the bark is cut in small pieces and boiled, it is removed and chewed and chewed until all the dye is removed and spit into a container. It is believed the saliva acts as a mordant to set the color.

Green Alder is known as **GIIST**, by Gitksan. The root and bark is decocted six hours for cough medicine. The pistillate catkins are a physic made by crushing the catkins and eating them when one is sleepy and thin.

For gonorrhea, both pistillate catkins and bark shavings were boiled and taken three times daily, working as a strong diuretic.

Natives of New Brunswick boiled stems until the bark came off, then chewed and swallowed the juice for lung hemorrhage, and to promote healing of fractures, and wounds.

The Mohawk used a decoction of alder twigs and couch grass root for "thick" urine.

Gray alder green cones were decocted to treat venereal disease in men, and as a wash for sore eyes. A root decoction was used by Seneca to treat burns, scalds and menstrual cramps.

Strong root decoctions were painted on traps for various animals, helping disguise the scent of humans.

Another interesting use was adding four dried, powdered bees to a root decoction for eye disease.

The early Acadian settlers brewed a reddish-brown tonic from the bark, to prevent anemia, and to treat kidney and skin complaints. Bark decoctions give a natural looking brown rinse to white or gray hair. In parts of Newfoundland, bark infusions are used for skin itching and rheumatism, or oil infused salves are applied to burns.

Herbal books of the 1600s suggested the use of fresh leaves for dissolving tumours. In 1973, a study into the properties of *Alnus oregona* verified that the stem bark contains lupeol and betulin, two compounds that suppress tumor activity. Sheth K et al, *Journal Pharm Sci* 62:1.

Charcoal made from alder was used in Europe for gunpowder. It makes a charcoal highly prized by artists. River alder charcoal was mixed with pitch by boreal natives to seal canoe seams. Bark decoctions were used to soak toboggan boards to soften them for bending and shaping.

A parasitic plant that grows near the root of Green Alder, or Spruce shows strong free radical scavenging activity. Poque, or Northern Ground Cone (*Boschniakia rossica*) contains various iridoid glucosides, and several other compounds of interest. It is occasionally found near birch, willow, and even leather leaf. Grizzly bears sometimes like to gorge on the thick, fleshy plants, which can be abundant in the floodplain cottonwood forests of northern valleys. In Alberta, it is most commonly found in the northern Caribou Mountains; but is somewhat rare.

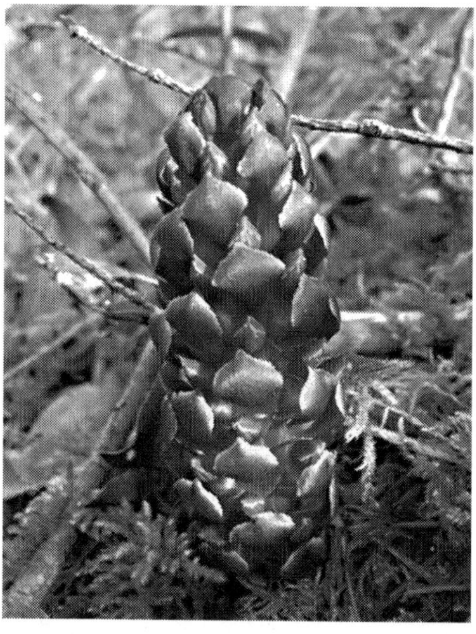

Poque
(Courtesy of Deborah Freeman)

The plants can grow for 4-5 years as an underground tuber, before flowering.

The name Poque probably originates from **P'UKW'ES**, the name given to the parasitic plant by the Kwakwaka'wakw.

The Slave tribe drank decoctions of the thick base stem for stomach aches.

The Gwich'in call this plant **DU'IINAHSHEE**, meaning "uncle's plant". They took the white core at the base of the plant and ground it into a powder, or simply chewed it for medicine. The powder could be combined with fat for skin rashes. The white middle part was boiled and eaten to increase appetite or relieve stomachaches.

It was called "pipe", as the wet, bulb-like underground portion was dried and a hole cut in to make a pipe. This was filled with dried willow leaves. Or the ground cone roots were dried, pounded and mixed with tobacco.

Studies in Poland show pollen extracts from alder increased survival rate of mice injected with acetaminophen.

Speckled or smooth alder is identified by its distinct visible triangular pith in a cross section of the stem. The leaf tea was used as a skin wash for pimples and a tonic, according to Seton. The bark and cones were used by the Inuit to dye reindeer and caribou skins.

River Alder is distributed from Alaska to western Saskatchewan; where the nearly identical Speckled Alder continues onto Atlantic Canada. River Alder may be simply a regional variation.

Sitka Alder is found in the extreme southwest part of Alberta, near Waterton National Park, but throughout British Columbia and north. Its uses are similar to above.

MEDICINAL

CONSTITUENTS- *A. crispa* bark- tannins, oils, resins, emodin, alnulin, protoalnulin, beta sitosterol, pinocembrin and phlobaphenes.
A. crispa- resins from buds and catkins (30-60%), pinosylvin and its methyl ether, pinostrobin and 2-phenethyl cinnamate, alpha and beta amyrin, betulin, lupeol, sterols.
A. incana bark- triterpenoids alnin-canone,taraxerol, salicin, and taraxerone.
Buds- betuletol, mikanin, quercitin, iso-rhamnetin, and 4'-6-7trimethyl-pectolinarigenin scutellarein.

Buds- ayanin, 3'-4'-5-trihydroxy-3-7-dimethoxy flavone, and 4'-5-dihydroxy-3-7-dimethoxy flavone, and genkwanin, quercitin, benzenoid 4'-5'-dihydroxy-3'-methoxy stilbene.

Both the leaves and dried inner bark of alder are bitter, helping stimulate digestion. Decoctions of the dried bark are astringent and hemostatic, reducing inflammations and even stopping internal hemorrhage. The powdered bark is a good hemostat for external bleeding. The fresh bark is emetic, and may cause cramping and vomiting.

Decoctions make an effective gargle for sore throats, pharyngitis, and toothaches. Milder dilutions cleanse teeth but also help to tighten and strengthen abscessed gums.

Work by Ritch-Krc et al, at College of New Caledonia in Prince George, BC found Mountain Alder (*A. incana*) possesses anti-cancer activity against mouse mastocytoma cells, with an IC50 value of only 6 ug/ml. *J Ethnopharm* 1996 52 151-6.

He mentions the case of an 11 year-old boy diagnosed with leukemia by a medical doctor in town of Vanderhoof. Sophie Thomas kept the boy at her home for a month and successfully treated him with *Alnus incana*. She also treated a young native woman with cervical cancer using alder and willow species.

Earlier studies found *A. crispa* extracts possess activity against gram-positive bacteria.

The inner bark of *A. incana ssp. rugosa* is a partial agonist of PPAR gamma activity, suggesting use in obesity and metabolic disease. Martineau et al, *Planta Med* 2010 13. Oregonin was identified as an inhibitor of adipogenesis in volume 14.

Pinocembrin, found in poplar and scullcap species, is active against *Bacillus subtilis, Candida albicans, Saccharcervisine species* and *Cryptococcus neoformans.*

Work in Poland by Gryzbek et al, found water extracts of *A. incana* cones have an inhibiting effect on HIV-1 reverse transcriptase. Both the stipes and cones, when extracted with ethyl acetate were found to exhibit weak activity against the D6 and W2 clones of *Plasmodium falciparum,* implicated in malaria.

Janice Schofield gives a recipe for diarrhea, using the unripe, green cones in decoction internally. (See below)

Externally, a useful wash can be made for various skin conditions including eczema, impetigo, poison ivy, bee stings, and various itching rashes.

Work by Webster et al, *J Ethnopharm* 2008 115:1 found mild anti-fungal activity from alder and giant goldenrod, and significant activity from strawberry, fireweed and *Potentilla simplex*.

David Winston, RH (AHG) writes, "Alder bark is considered a specific for skin conditions where the eruptions (pimples) are red, raised, and never come to a head. It can be used orally, and topically for boils, carbuncles, staph infections, and large painful pimples on back, buttocks, face or neck".

Ellingwood noted similar benefits, as well as improvement in gastric secretions and improved digestion.

A good combination for pustular psoriasis is equal parts of alder bark, Oregon grape root and yellow dock root.

When available fresh, the slimy cambium layer can be rubbed over skin conditions, for even better effect.

Alder's primary use is to improve nutrition, by increasing digestion and the rate of waste excretion. Like poplar and willow, the bark of alder contains salicin, but in lesser amounts. Lupeol, is found in both alder and birch.

Catkins, from Red Alder (*A. rubra*), common throughout British Columbia, showed significant anti-fungal activity against all nine species studied; the catkins more so than the bark. McCutcheon et al, *Journal Ethnopharm* 1994 44:3.

Anti-microbial activity was found by same authors for bark and catkins, with nine of nine species showing some degree of inhibition. *J Ethnopharm* 1992 37.

Both *A. incana* and *A. viridis* bark are cytotoxic to HeLa cancer cells. A dry extract of the cones is anti-microbial. Stevic et al, *J Med Food* 2010 13:3.

Alnus incana bark has been found, *in vitro*, to inhibit CYP3A4 enzyme activity in the liver and hence delay breakdown of various prescription drugs; at least in theory. Tam et al, *Can J Physio Pharmacol* 2011 89:1.

Altan, obtained from cones of Black Alder (*A. glutinosa*) exhibits hepatoprotective activity at 1 mg/kg, which is about ten times less than traditional flavonoid-based medicines.

The green cones may be tinctured and used for allergies, as well as bacteria, fungal and amoebic infections. The freshly dried green cones, catkins, leaves and twigs can be tinctured for moving blood and lymph.

Kiva Rose, noted herbalist, writes: "Alder is a staple of my clinical work and one of my most beloved herbal allies. Its consistent and powerful ability to act as a profound alterative and lymphatic while addressing even the most severe microbial infections makes it truly invaluable to almost any practitioner."

She notes alder does not add to fluids or move or contain them, but transforms their quality.

She continues. "I have repeatedly seen cases of staph (including several confirmed cases of MRSA) infection manifesting as repeated outbreaks of boils clear up with the consistent use of Alder tincture."

Combine with Oregon grape root for constipation with poor fat digestion and skin problems.

Boggy congested conditions call for alder and bogbean, or perhaps Spanish Needles (*Bidens tripartita*) if the pattern suits.

Small amounts of tincture in ice-cold water will help move congested lymph, swollen glands and chronic sore throats.

Combine with redroot for severe lymphatic congestion, and with wild bergamot or calendula when a warming stimulant for circulation is needed.

Tag Alder (*A. serrulata*) is used for chronic skin conditions, lymphatic stagnation, dyspepsia in the elderly, and external hemorrhoids.

The leaves are a suitable substitute for plantain in cases of insect bites, bee stings, and assorted thorns, splinters and wilderness nicks and scrapes.

The leaf of the related *A. hirsuta* contains hirsutanonol, a compound that blocks LPS- and IFN-γ-induced macrophage iNOS expression.

Alnustic acid, derived from leaves of related *A. firma* inhibits HIV. Yu et al, *Arch Pharm Res* 30:7.

The leaves of *A. japonica* possess anti-inflammatory compounds. Han et al, *J Ag Food Chem* 2008 56:1.

NOTE- The fresh bark is griping and can be emetic or cathartic. Use dried bark. Fresh green cones can be tinctured as soon as possible. Chop well.

HOMEOPATHY

Red Alder is a close relative used as a remedy for skin afflictions, sub-maxillary glandular enlargements, and poor digestion due to insufficient secretion of gastric juices.

It stimulates nutrition and soothes ulcerated membranes of throat and mouth.

In the female, it may be used for vaginal discharge, cervical dysplasia, or where there is easy bleeding. It will help bring on delayed menstruation when the pain is from the back towards the pubic area.

In chronic herpes infection of the skin, or poison ivy it may be used locally.

DOSE- Tincture to the third potency.

GEMMOTHERAPY

EUROPEAN ALDER
(*A. glutinosa*)

This is the remedy for all chronic, inflammatory conditions. It is for all patients with coronary conditions, arthritis, pleuro-pneumonia, peritonitis, osteomyelitis, and staph infections. It is also for the early stages of acute articular rheumatism, coronary thrombosis, mitral stenosis, Paget's disease, osteoporosis, Consequently this is a global hypo coagulant, hypo-viscosant and anti-thrombosis bud therapy.

Use in resolution stage after infarction or other vascular spasms, phlebitis, acute or chronic migraines associated with cerebral circulation.

Take at first stage of flu, sinusitis, tracheitis.

Use for colitis, peritonitis and cholecystitis.

Use in cases of chronic urticaria, as well as kidney issues such as cystitis and pyelitis.

MOUNTAIN/RIVER ALDER
(*A. incana*)

The action is similar to the European species but is stronger and shorter acting in nature. It has the ability to reduce severe inflammatory and thrombosis conditions, but must be used more often in smaller doses.

DOSE- 15-20 drops in water three times daily. European Alder once daily. Both are 1 DH glycerine macerates. *Alnus incana* buds contain quinic and ferulic acid.

NORTHERN GROUNDCONE
POQUE
(*Boschniakia rossica* [Cham & Schltdl] B. Fedtsch**)**
(*B. glabra* CA Mey ex Bong**)**

CONSTITUENTS- Two iridoid glucosides, boschnaloside and boschnaside, an oligosaccaride (+)-pinoresinol-beta-D-glucopyranoside, and rossicasides A & G-K, phenylpropanoid glycosides, have been isolated. Orobanin of an iridoid glucoside and the pyridine alkaloids of boschniaside, boschnilactone and boschniakine have been identified.

Boschniakia is named after the Russian amateur botanist A. K. Boschniak.

Boschniakia is a brown to yellow to red parasitic plant found near Green Alder (*A. crispa*) and other *Alnus* species. It is commonly found at the foot of trees looking like an upright pinecone, about 20 cm long, with dense dark flowers and a dark scale-like leaf below it. At first glance they appear dead, but are fresh and resilient when touched. It belongs to the Broomrape family.

The Tlingit of Alaska use *B. glabra* root as part of a treatment for sores. The Dena'ina of Alaska call it **QINAZ'IN**, "that which sticks up". A piece of the plant was tied around the neck of puppies or babies to help them grow correctly. It is said to be a favourite food of bears.

In Japan, the dried herb, or stems are used as a tonic. Research conducted by Tsuda et al, in Japan in 1994, found *B. rossica* to possess strong free radical scavenging activity, and therefore, strong inhibitory effect on disorders caused by free radical damage.

Piao et al, *Zhong Xi Yi He Xue Bao* 2003 1:2 found extracts clear free radicals for D-galactose-induced senile rats.

Wu et al, *World J Gastroenterol* 2005 11:1 found extracts prevent pig serum-induced liver rat fibrosis by inhibiting the activation of hepatic stellate cells and synthesizing collagen.

Poque has been found to protect ECly hepatic cells by reducing oxidative stress, suppressing inflammation and improved CYP2E1 detoxification of liver. Quan et al, *Biosci Biotech Biochem* 2009 73:4. Inhibition of triglycerides in HepG2 cells has been noted. Zhang et al, *Fitoterapia* 2013 85:69-75. Both mitochondria and death receptor mediated apoptosis pathways are involved in anti-tumor potential of a polysaccharide in Hep2 larynx cancer cell lines. Wang Z et al, *Gene* 2014 536:1.

In Jilin province, China, *B. rossica* is used as an anti-senile agent. Ethanol extracts were administered to rats whose cholinergic nucleus had been destroyed by ibotenic acid. Rats treated with the extract showed significant improvement in learning ability, and it was concluded *B. rossica* would be therapeutic in the treatment of senility.

In Traditional Chinese Medicine, the herb is known as **JOU-TSUNG-JUNG**, for it's nutritious but not harsh qualities, as well as ease and smoothness.

It is considered a sweet, salty flavor with warming properties; affecting the kidney and large intestine.

It nourishes the kidneys and sperm, supplements yang, and moistens the intestines. It has been used for impotence, infertility in women, and cold obstructions of the loins and knees. Pharmacological studies show toning and laxative effect. It increases saliva secretions in laboratory mice and shows hypotensive effect from both water and alcohol soluble extracts.

The parasitic plant contains three compounds that induce the excitable catnip response in cats. These are boschniakine, boschnialactone, and onikulactone. It is possible the scent was used to attract and trap larger cats by native hunters of the coast.

Boschniakine is found in various species of *Pedicularis*, the semi-parasitic Lousewort.

BARK/LEAF OIL

Combine one part of freshly dried bark and leaves to five parts canola oil in a low temperature crock pot for six hours. Strain and use as part of anti-inflammatory salves or ointments, or indolent slow-healing skin ulcers. It combines well with goldenrod and Artemisia plant oils for strained or injured tissue, with arnica and St. John's wort for nerve and muscle pain, and with wild bergamot or cleaver oil for inflamed, swollen glands.

HYDROSOL

Upon distillation of the green leaves, catkins and twigs of alder, a hydrosol is obtained. Dr. Ayer recommended the use of *Alnus* water for periodic hyperasthetic rhinitis (hay-fever). The hydrosol is combined with an equal amount of water and snuffed up the nostrils 5-6 times, or atomized at full strength into the nose.

At night the water is combined with un-petroleum jelly and smeared into the nose; while the distillate is taken internally, one teaspoon three times daily one hour before or after meals to improve digestion.

Dr. Ayer also recommended this as a cure in the acute stage of gonorrhea, or as an antidote to poison ivy skin rashes.

The hydrosol is produced when catkins are forming, using bark and catkins.

WAX

Psylla wax is secreted by an aphid (*Prociphilus alni*), living on leaves of River Alder (*Alnus incana*). It is obtained by extracting it from the insects first in hot ether, in order to remove the glycerides, and then with hot chloroform.

The wax is insoluble in hot ether, and only poorly soluble in cold chloroform. It crystallizes in needles with a silky luster; and melts at 96 degrees Celsius.

Psylla wax is the psyllostearylic acid of psyllostearyl alcohol.

No commercial use at present time.

The aphids cover themselves with wax, secreted by their bodies. They have an interesting relationship with the Green Lacewing (*Chrysopa spp.*)

Their larvae are the same size and shape as aphids, which they love to puncture and suck dry.

The aphids produce honey nectar for ants that protect them like milk cows. Lacewing larvae protect themselves by stripping the wax off their prey and piling it on themselves.

It adheres very well to their bristly hooked body, fooling ants into thinking they are aphids. When stripped of the wax, it takes them only about twenty minutes to go back into disguise.

FLOWER ESSENCES

Green alder flower essence helps to open our hearts and minds to aspects of light which are beyond normal perception. This relaxation and expansion of our sensory awareness allows us to access subtle levels of information from our surroundings. It helps us integrate this level so that we may see beyond our current habits and belief systems. **ALASKA**

Alder flower essence is for acceptance of our destiny, and the anger and blame, including self-blame, and lack of energy and joy that comes from acceptance of self. With the essence, we learn to forgive ourselves and learn about spiritual protection in disputes. **OGAM**

Essence of Alder is associated with the principle of release. It reduces stress, anxiety, and nervousness and increases life energy. **GIFFORD**

Speckled Alder (*A. incana*) essence is for stepping out of habitual patterns, enabling on to listen to instinct and take responsibility. It helps release energy deficiency, victim mentality and not learning from mistakes. **ICELANDIC**

River Alder (*A. incana*) essence helps relax groups and work with colleagues. **MIRIAM**

Alder essence is for taking life at surface value; being unable to see what one senses to be true; helps us to integrate seeing with knowing so that we can recognize our highest truth in each life experience.
DARCY WILLIAMSON

Poque is the remedy for claustrophobia—enables us to survive in close quarters, to maintain self in closed area, cities, apartments. Also assists when feeling too much going on around us. Feeling closed in by demands. **FREEMAN & MONGEAU**

SPIRITUAL PROPERTIES

Red Alder energy has a quality of innocent, child-like enthusiasm that is both stimulating and cheerful. It offers an outpouring of energy that insists that you get on with life and open your eyes to the beauty around you. Seek out red alder when you feel depressed, overly serious, or find yourself dwelling on the past. Red Alder turns up the music, sets your toes to tapping, and before you know it, you are dancing into the future. **CHASE/PAWLIK**

The alder reminds us of the need to blend strength and courage with generosity of spirit and compassion. There is a time to challenge things and a time to hold our peace. The alder teaches us this discrimination and the need to see beneath the surface of things. **GIFFORD**

PERSONALITY TRAITS

The flames of Alder are green, but its blood is red. Alder is the bleeding mother and the wounded healer who understands; it is the listener, who can listen to your sorrow and weave your tears into her life-giving carpet.

Master of the elements, Alder can heal with water, fire, earth and air.
HAGENEDER

Alder is an excellent magical name for one who is secretive, changeable, a fire sign; one who loves color; a seamstress or an artist; one who loves incense, aftershave lotion or perfume; a down-to-earth person who is a forest lover and a wise experienced Witch.

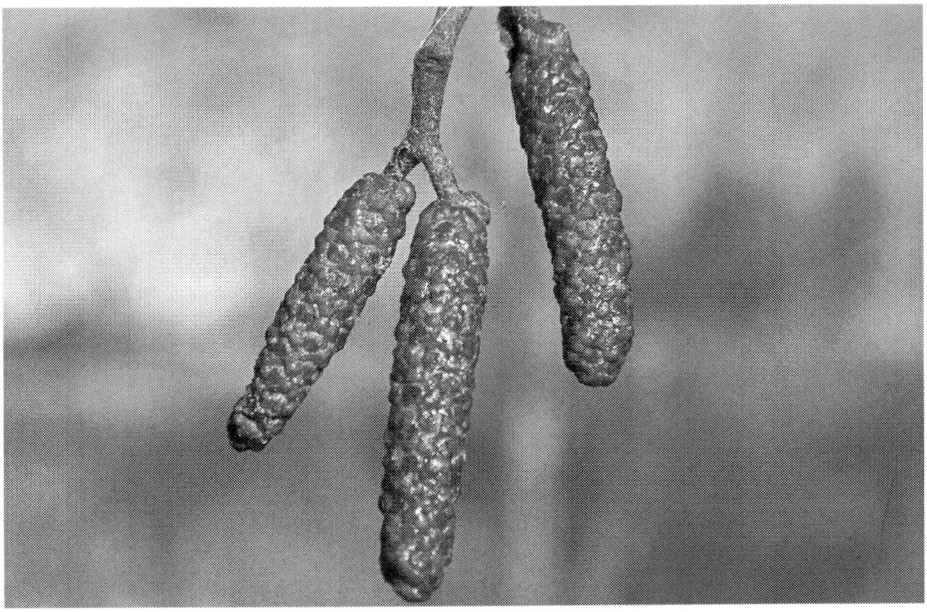

Green Alder catkins

This is the sort of person who loves the drams of ritual, who likes to dance skyclad in the shadows of the forest. Alder will bring out the hidden sensitivity and sentimentality lurking within you.

MCFARLAND

If the patient is healthy on the emotional level, the only characteristic personality trait may be his tendency to generosity. One would not normally consider "having a kind heart" to be a symptom, but in the case of Alnus it is something that is at the centre of the patient's being.

He or she is willing to make sacrifices for others and to do favours, which, for most other people, would not be possible.

As this type of behaviour often brings its own day-to-day rewards, there may not be a noticeable loss of vitality in the patient.

Many remedies have the feeling of being isolated and alone. Alnus is unique in their reaction to this feeling of isolation in that, in order to overcome it, they may tell the practitioner: "I try harder and work harder as I easily feel guilt. Also, I have a tremendous natural sympathy for others, especially for those people who have less or who are suffering in some way."

They deny that they have needs; therefore, they postpone gratification and then eventually they suffer from not having their emotional and physical nourishment needs met. They can become resentful, bitter and empty; then later, in theory, they might "gorge" themselves emotionally, taking more than they need from life.

In the third stage, depression becomes constant and then, finally, they start to become apathetic, as if all the previous caring had been "burned" out of them. Eventually they develop a complete indifference to life. At the end of this stage, when they hate life, they hate other people for being so selfish. **OLSEN**

MYTHS AND LEGENDS

According to legend, at the time of Creation, there was a rivalry between God and the devil. The wolf was shaped by God, but the devil tried to intervene and bring it to life.

However, the wolf refused to breathe and live. It was only when infused with the power of God that the wolf sprang to life and began to attack the devil. The devil hid in an alder tree but the wolf caught hold of his heal (sic) and blood ran down the trunk. From that time forward, the alder has had its reddish bark. **KNAB**

According to one such tale, mink-man, a primordial human-animal figure of the Distant Time, approached a group of human-plant figures known as tree-women...His solemn duty was to inform the tree-women that Raven, the sacred transformer spirit who happened to also be husband to each of the tree-women, had just died. Upon hearing this sad news, each of the tree-women expressed her profound sorrow by inflicting a superficial flesh wound to her body...One of the grieving tree-women was transformed into an alder [and] she cried and pinched herself until she bled...her distinctively colored bark oozed a blood red juice, which the Koyukon traditionally used as a red dye.

KNUDTSON/SUZUKI

The medieval Wulfdietrich Saga gives a strong idea of Alder Woman. In various German legends she appears to wanderers as a seductive woman teaching wanton males a lesson by turning into a hairy or bark-like creature once in their embrace.

Her different German names—Else, Elsa, Elise—are derived from the Anglo-Saxon Alor, or the Gothic Alisa...

In the second song of the Wulfdietrich, Saga the Rough Else, a wild-looking woman of the woods who is covered in hair, puts a spell on the hero eventually making him made. He runs wildly through the woods, living on herbs for six months. Then she takes him on a ship over the sea to another land where she is queen.

She bathes in a magical well that washes away her rough skin, and is transformed into the most beautiful of women and has a new name—Sigeminne (victory of love). **HAGENEDER**

An old European legend about the origin of alders is related to April 21st, the festival day of the goddess Pales. She was the Roman goddess of shepherds and herdsmen.

Two men decided to spend the holiday fishing, instead of attending the required ceremonies. In punishment, the goddess turned them both into trees destined forever to haunt the banks of streams, watching for fish.

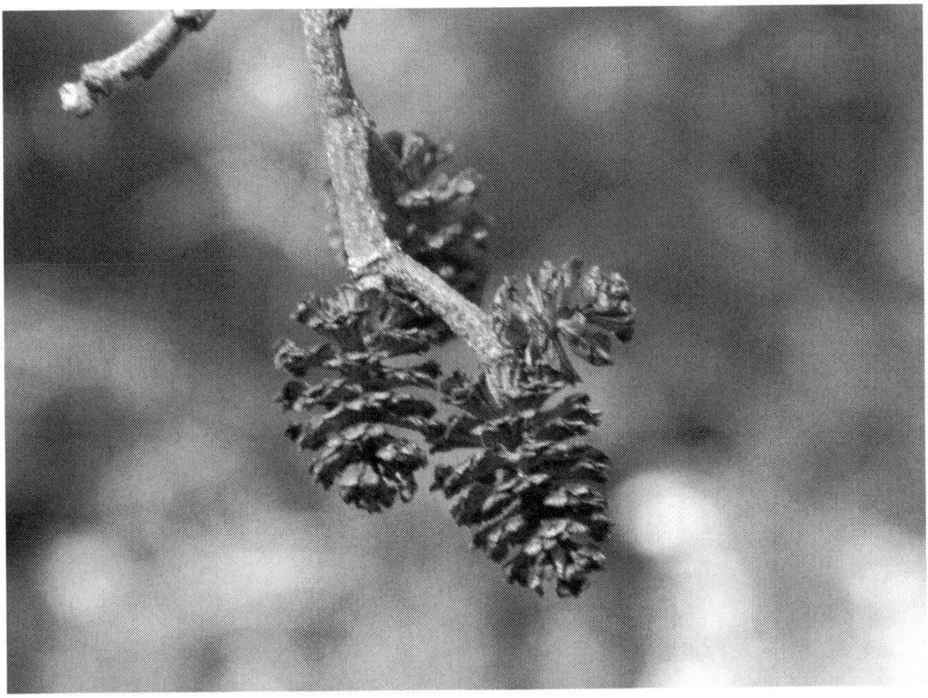

Dry Brown Alder cone

RECIPES

INFUSION- To one ounce of fresh or dried bark add one pint of boiling water. Let steep 20 minutes. Take 1-2 tablespoons as needed.

DECOCTION- Take one ounce of green, unripe female cones and simmer in one pint of water for twenty minutes. Drink as needed. (Janice Schofield)

Decoct the dried bark (1:20) for improving food absorption and fat metabolism. Take one to two ounces before meals. Also good for throat gargles, gum weakness, etc.

TINCTURE- 5-20 drops, as needed. For pustular psoriasis, as noted above, 25 drops three times daily in cool water for 4-6 months. A tincture is made from the dried, green cones, and twigs at 1:5 and 40% alcohol. Use for intestinal inflammation.

SALVE- Cover one part fresh-stripped alder bark with five parts coconut oil in a glass jar. Let sit in sun for two weeks, shaking daily. If inclement weather, use low temperature crockpot. Strain and use for skin conditions such as eczema and psoriasis.

SYRUP- Macerate three pounds of crushed dry bark in cold water for six hours. Put into percolator and add water until five pints have passed over. Put on low heat and stir in eight pounds of honey or sugar. When cold, add a pint of whiskey or vodka.

B. rossica- 6-18 grams. For treating constipation, 12-18 grams dry powder.

BITTERSWEET VINE
FALSE BITTERSWEET
AMERICAN BITTERSWEET
WAXWORK
STAFF VINE
FEVER TWIG
(*Celastrus scandens* L.)
ORIENTAL BITTERSWEET
(*C. orbiculatus* Thunb.)
PARTS USED- seed, bark and root bark

Celastrus is from the Greek **KELASTROS**, an ancient name of *Phillyrea latifolia*. Other authors believe it is from the Greek **KELAS**, meaning the latter season.

Bittersweet is a woody, perennial climber hardy to Zone 3. It produces bright yellow orange berries on the female, although both male and female plants are required for fruit to form. The fruit is not edible.

It twines around posts and trellises, and up house walls with assistance. The green leaves turn a bright yellow in fall. Bittersweet is sometimes confused with Dulcamara (*Solanum dulcamara*), hence the name False Bittersweet.

The plant was traditionally used for rheumatism, menstrual disorders and liver disorders, but is rarely used today.

Dr. King wrote it is an "alterative, diaphoretic and diuretic with some narcotic powers.

Use in scrofula, secondary syphilis, chronic hepatic affections, cutaneous affections, leucorrhea, rheumatism and obstructed menstruation. Externally, an ointment has been successfully employed in inflamed and indurated breasts, in pruritis vulvae, burns, etc."

Rafinesque, back in 1830, considered False Bittersweet the equivalent of Dulcamara and Mezereum, but weaker in action.

Gunn wrote, "the bark of the root...has a sweetish and a rather sickening taste; it is both a powerful and useful medicine, although like most of the valuable medicinal plants of our country...its virtues are but little known or appreciated...It increases all the secretions and excretions, particularly perspiration; acts gently as a diuretic, or increases the flow of urine. It is highly regarded in liver complaints, and in all general weakness."

William Cook suggested the plant is "very good, combined with mild tonics, for young women about the age of puberty, when they get blue bands under their eyes, with general paleness, precarious appetite, nervousness, feebleness and vaginal weakness. I have obtained a good impression from it in some mild cases of chronic ovaritis."

The Fox combined mullein leaves before flowering, with coltsfoot leaves (*Petasites palmata*) and the root of bittersweet for tuberculosis. They used it in a compound medicine for, "relief of women in labour".

The Chippewa used stalk decoctions for skin eruptions, and root decoctions for urine retention.

The Ojibwa called it **MANIDOBIMA' KWIT**, and used the inner bark in winter soups. The vine and bark are emergency food. Like *Aralia nudicaulis* it is associated with the rabbit due to its value as famine food.

The Cherokee used strong compound infusion, with red raspberry leaves for the pain of childbirth.

They chewed the bark for coughs, and the thorny branches for rubbing rheumatism. The leaves are highly astringent, and infused for bowel complaints. Infusions of bark were used to settle stomachs, while stronger decoctions were for the bowel, skin eruptions or the stoppage of urine.

The roots were boiled and made into an ointment for cancerous and indolent skin ulcers and sores.

The Creek tribe used the plant for women with urinary trouble or pain in the small of the back.

The Iroquois decocted the roots and gave it to young girls who catch cold and don't menstruate. The leaves and stems were infused to promote regular menstruation, as a diuretic, and to reduce fevers and soreness from pregnancy.

The orange berries are often sold at roadside stands throughout the Appalachians, for flower arranging.

In China, the closely related *C. orbiculatus,* or **NAN SHE T'ENG** is used medicinally for its warming properties that help relieve inflammation and detoxify the body. It stimulates blood circulation to open up meridian passageways, expels gas and strengthens the sinews and bones.

It is often used in cases of paralysis with numbness of extremities, headaches, toothache, and spontaneous abscess formation. The leaves stems and root are all used in decoction; while the leaves are crushed and applied to external conditions as a poultice.

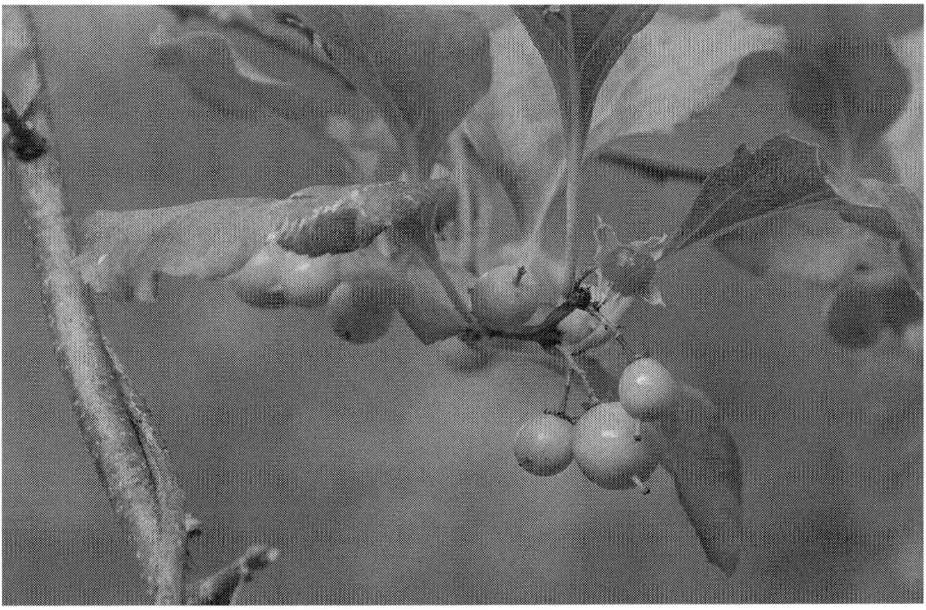

American Bittersweet

C. orbiculatus is hardy to zone 2B in the United States, and would probably grow on the prairies in a protected spot. In trials at Morden, it grew well with a hardiness of 6.6.

In India, the related *C. paniculatus*, or **JYOTISMATI**, is used in Ayurvedic medicine for promoting intellect, as well as curing ulcers and pustular eruptions of the skin.

The flowers are analgesic and anti-inflammatory. Ahmad et al, *Journal of Ethnopharmacology* May 1994.

The seed oil contains celapinine, and is a stimulant for both rheumatic and paralytic pain.

The seed oil has anti-fertility activity, according studies by Bidwai reported in same journal in 1990. The leaf juice is used as an antidote for opium poisoning.

MEDICINAL

CONSTITUENTS- tannins, celastrol (a yellow quinode nortriterpene); celaxanthin (carotenoid), celastine, volatile oils, tannins.

False Bittersweet was a major component of the Compound Scrophularia syrup, an important cancer formula of Eclectic physicians. It was considered without equal for removing liver obstructions.

The green leaves were valued, by Eli Jones, as an ointment to treat breast cancer.

It is a strong alterative that helps move morbid wastes and toxins from the body. Dr. Cook recommends the root for glandular swellings, combining best with Moonseed (Yellow Parilla), Yellow Dock, and Gentian root.

He considers this suitable not only for scrofula, but for various scaly skin conditions.

"It is very good, combined with mild tonics, for young women about the age of puberty, when they get blue bands under their eyes, with general paleness, precarious appetite, nervousness, feebleness and vaginal weakness. I have obtained a good impression from it in some mild cases of chronic ovaritis... I have found it good in the enuresis of nervous children, generally combining it with agrimonia.

Outwardly, a strong decoction...makes a good wash in chaffiness of the skin and scaly eruptions, especially when the surface is hot.

It is used in poultices, salve and a strong decoction with flannel upon glandular swellings, and has a soothing and softening action."

Matthew Wood adds. "Celastrus acts on the small intestine to improve absorption and nutrition. It is indicated in wasting, or withering, but also in congestion and edema due to weakness of the lymphatic vessels surrounding the intestines and kidneys. It is even beneficial in diabetes insipidus and bedwetting, not as an astringent, but by nourishing the parts to retain fluids. Cook used it in combination with agrimony for enuresis in delicate, nervous children."

Matthew believes, "it definitely has an influence on the endocrine system, the adrenocortical situation, and sex hormones. It probably has an effect on the hypothalamus."

Dr. Carey used a strong ointment for hemorrhoids for over 15 years on a variety of patients.

The root bark of Bittersweet shows evidence of both anti-bacterial and anti-fungal activity. In the past, the root bark has been used for its calming effects and to induce menstruation, when delayed.

In studies conducted by Heisey and Gorham at Fordham University in New York (1992); Bittersweet root bark showed activity against *Streptococcus mutans, Trichophyton rubrum* and *Candida albicans.*

It is strongly active against *E. coli.* Hayes et al, *Bot Gaz* 1947 108.

The root and bark have diuretic effect.

In 1951, a US patent was granted for root use as a non-toxic food preservative.

The fruit, combined with lard, gives a golden salve that is mild and soothing. The root bark salve may be used topically for liver spots, obstinate sores, skin cancer, eruptions and tumors.

Sesquiterpenes from *C. orbiculatus* roots have been found more active than verpamil in reversing vinblastine resistance in multi-drug-resistant KB-VI cells. Kim et al, *J of Natural Products* 1998 61:1.

It has been used for treating rheumatoid arthritis and bacterial infections. Anti-tumor activity has been reported.

FRUIT OIL

The oil from the fruit of *Celastrus paniculatus* is known as Dukudu oil, and used for rheumatism and for religious observance in India and Sri Lanka.

SEED OIL

In 1932, the oil from the red seeds of *C. scandens*, gathered in Kentucky showed substantial quantities of the esters of formic, acetic and later, benzoic acid. There are four to six the size of grape seeds in each fruit.

When ground and extracted with ethyl ether, it yielded 47% fatty oil; and with petroleum ether about 36%.

The seed oil is composed of mostly linolenic (39%) and linoleic acids (45%); as well as 12% palmitic and traces of stearic and oleic acids.

The oil has a saponification value of 297, iodine number of 121.5, and acid value of 3.9.

It contains 17.6 hexabromides; soluble fatty acids like butyric acid 19%, with 2.96 un-saponifiables.

The seed oil of *C. paniculatus* has been shown to improve the memory and learning in rats. Norepinephrine, dopamine, serotonin, and their metabolites were all noted to decline. Researchers contend this represents a decrease in monoamine turnover.

Other researchers confirm the oils positive effect on memory, and found that it did not act via acetylcholine, but they did find evidence of activity on central muscarinic sites.

SPIRITUAL PROPERTIES

To help you forget about an unhappy love affair, place a sprig of Bittersweet under your bed. Traditionally, Bittersweet was used to remove spells and hexes. Wearing some around your neck will alleviate dizziness and help you stay focused. **SUSAN GREGG**

MYTHS AND LEGENDS

This is one of the Winabojo remedies, the native name being Winabojo onagic, meaning "Winabojo's intestines". The legend is that Winabojo was once walking on the ice when he heard something rattling behind him. He looked back and saw that his intestines were dragging behind him and part had become frozen to the ice. He broke off part and threw them over a tree, saying, "This shall be for the good of my future relatives". **CHIPPEWA LEGEND**

PERSONALITY TRAITS

Psychologically, it helps people with weak boundaries, who get wrapped up in other people's problems. **WOOD**

Celastraceae can enhance community living, but it can also drive people apart. Rather than experiencing life with the solitary introversion of a dull mind, weak body and irritable nature, one can join society with friendliness, lively communication, mental acumen, physical stamina and even exaltation of spirits. One must just make sure the exhilaration does not go too far, resulting in a depletion that can merely allow for a solitary existence. **VERMUELEN**

RECIPES

DECOCTION- 2-4 ounces three times daily.

EXTRACT- 5-10 grains

TINCTURE- 1-3 drops per dose.

OINTMENT- Take one pound of fresh green leaves to two pounds of lard and one ounce of beeswax. Simmer, and strain. Rub into the breast twice daily for tumours.

ROOT OINTMENT- Take one part of fresh root to one part of lard and gently simmer for several hours. Remove from heat and add beeswax to harden. Coconut oil may be substituted to help form anal suppositories to treat hemorrhoids.

CAUTION- Do not use internally during pregnancy, lactation, with bradycardia or concurrently with digitalis-like alkaloids. Do not exceed traditional dosage and do not use long term as a simple. Do not use fruit internally.

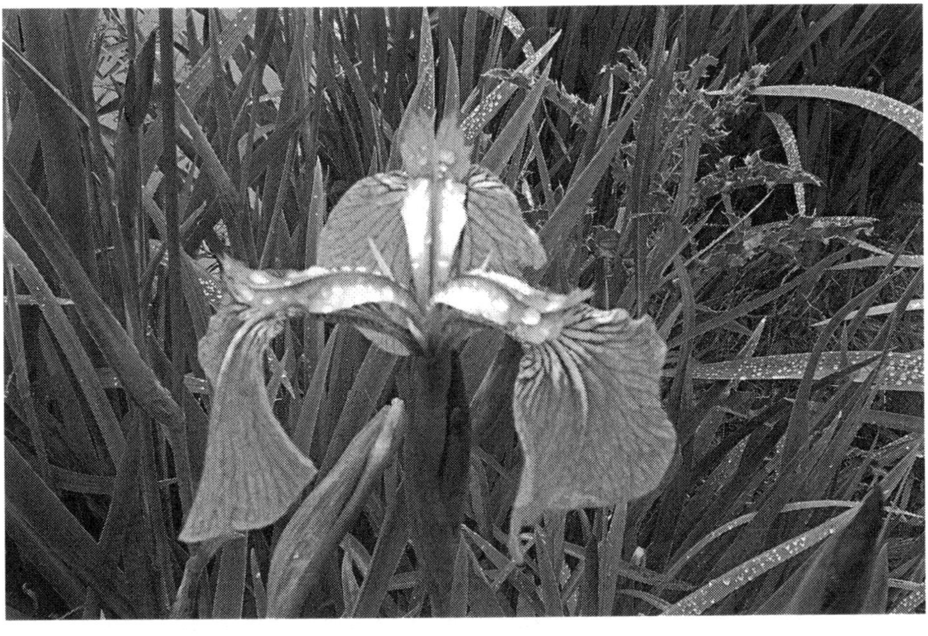

Western Blue Flag

NORTHERN BLUE FLAG
(*Iris versicolour* L.)
WESTERN BLUE FLAG
ROCKY MOUNTAIN IRIS
(*I. missouriensis* Nutt.)
BEARDED IRIS
GERMAN IRIS
(*I. germanica* L.)
FLORENTINE IRIS
ORRIS IRIS
(*I. germanica* L. var. *florentina* Dykes)
FLEUR-DE-LIS
SIBERIAN IRIS
(*I. sibirica* L.)
DALMATIAN IRIS
(*I. pallida* Lam.)
YELLOW FLAG
WATER FLAG
(*I. pseudacorus* L.)
NORTH CHINA IRIS
(*I. pallasii var. chinensis* Fisch. ex Trevir)
OREGON IRIS
(*I. tenax* Dougl. ex Lind)
PARTS USED- rhizome, flower

Blue Flags, yellow flags, flags all freckled
Which will you take? Yellow, blue, speckled!
Take which you will, speckled, blue, yellow,
Each in its way has not a fellow. **C. ROSSETTI**

If someone may assume that the iris at midnight sways and bends,
Attempting to focus the North Star
Exactly at the blue-tinged center of its pale stem.
PATTIANN ROGERS

O fleur-de-luce, bloom on, and let the river
Linger to kiss thy feet;
O flower of song, bloom on, and make forever
The world more fair and sweet. **LONGFELLOW**

I am prepared; here is my keen-edged sword,
Decked with five Flower-de-luces on each side. **SHAKESPEARE**

Born in the purple, born to joy and pleasance
Thou dost not toil nor spin
But makest glad and radiant with thy presence
The meadow and the lin. **LONGFELLOW**

Iris is from the Greek word for rainbow. Orris is derived from the Italian Orice or Oris, from the middle Italian Irios. The Spanish word **ARCOIRIS**, Iris's Arch, means rainbow.

Tenax means tenacious, and named by David Douglas, due to the strength of the leaf fibre. Pseudoacorus means false acorus, or sweet flag. Versicolor is various-colored, and missouriensis means from Missouri.

In mythology, the Goddess Iris was Juno's personal messenger, who traveled over the rainbow to reach Earth. She probably began as a form of Kali-Maya, a pre-Vedic mistress of the rainbow who shifted reality through her cosmic veils. Iris was responsible for leading the souls of dead women to Elysian Fields, the Greek version of heaven.

At one time, it was thought that everything was based on rainbows, because strong sunlight would reveal millions of tiny rainbows.

In Virgil's Aeneid, Iris is sent to gather up the souls of women. She appears to the dying Queen Dido, and carries away a lock of the queen's hair in order to free her soul from her body.

The Egyptian Pharaohs topped their scepters with an iris design, the 3 petals representing wisdom, faith and courage. In ancient Greece, Iris was the name of both the female messenger of the gods and her bridge to earth, the rainbow. Both Greeks and Romans decorated tombs with iris depictions. Ancient Minoan frescoes in Crete, and 3500 year-old carvings on the walls of the great temple of Karnak, at Luxor, Egypt speak of the ancient reverence.

Because she carried all the bad news, and Hermes all the good, rainbows were originally a sign of foreboding.

According to one myth, Iris was one of Zeus's lovers, changed into a flower.

Iris was believed used medicinally in Egypt as far back as 1540 BC, when King Thutmose I had the flower drawn on the temple wall of Theban Ammon, at Karnak.

The root powder and juice were used as a cathartic and diuretic, to treat convulsions, coughs, upset stomach, insect bites and acne.

The first record of irises in gardens is from 1479 BC, when King Thutmose III conquered Syria. He took home, it is said, every flower he found in that country.

Bearded Iris (*I. germanica*) is a most ancient cultivated plant, domesticated nearly four millenium ago.

Medicine borrowed the name in 1721, when Danish anatomist Jacob Winslow applied the word iris to the human eye, after the varied colours observed. Iris is a bridge between the known and unknown.

White irises are traditionally planted on Muslim graves, to ensure prosperity in the next world. The three-part iris appears often in Islamic art, textiles, carvings and illustrations.

To the Chinese, iris is a symbol of grace, affection and beauty in solitude. In Japan, irises were placed on roofs to protect against fire, and purify the environment. May 5th is Iris Bathing Day, and leaf tea is added to bath water to protect one for next year.

Various iris roots are used in the West Indies, as seated voodoo dolls. Although associated with rainbows, a true bright red iris has yet to be hybridized.

Van Gogh's Irises, and Georgia O'Keeffe's Black Iris, are two famous paintings.

Missouri Flag, or Western Blue Flag is a widespread beard-less iris that grows wild from Mexico to southern Alberta, but ironically, not in Missouri. It is very frost hardy; with the flower colours varying from very pale blue to lavender, and even white. It is considered an endangered species in southern Alberta, and needs protection.

Noted Alberta herbalist Ruth Yanor suggests that good eco-terrorists make use of this endangered and protected status by planting it in wet areas on their land to discourage herbicide spraying near their residence. Makes sense to me, so I pass it on!

Western Blue Flag requires very special conditions of wet meadows in spring, but well-drained and drier environment by mid-summer.

Only two sites near Carway and Whiskey Gap contain significant numbers, and both are under significant stress from water drainage problems. At Whisky Gap, a site overgrazed by cattle and dry soil, the plants did not bloom for 25 years, until the wet summer of 1991.

Western Blue Flag has been found in Banff National Park and at one isolated location north of Calgary.

Agricultural pesticides used for "farm management" pose a serious threat to this plant.

Various native tribes, including the Paiute and Shoshone made great use of this plant. The ripe seeds were made into a paste and applied to body sores, or burns.

Warm root decoctions were dropped into the ears for earache, or drunk for stomach, bladder troubles and such.

The root was crushed and poulticed on skin sores, including impetigo, staph and venereal sores, or for soothing rheumatic pains. Small pieces were chewed for toothache, the root believed to kill the nerves and the tooth would come out.

Natives of New Mexico believed the fresh root to be poisonous, but sliced and threaded the dry root into necklaces. These were worn as protection from smallpox, as it closes the throat, and the necklace would help keep it open.

Iris missouriensis contains irisen in the rootstock, that when fresh, was mixed with animal bile as an arrow poison.

Wounded victims succumbed in 3-5 days from even the slightest exposure.

Northern Blue Flag has the greatest reputation, of all the irises, for medicinal purpose. It is mainly an Eastern species, but is native to Manitoba, and does creep into north-central Saskatchewan and Idaho.

The fiber from the outer edge of the leaves has been used to make rope, netting and fabric bags. It is tedious work, with twelve feet of rope taking up to six weeks work.

The Ojibwa name **WEEKAEHN** means, "that which extracts". Another name, **PAKWIASKO'NS** means, "waterweed".

Many native tribes planted Blue Flag or wild iris around ponds, just as the Northern Cree planted Calamus, so that it would be available wherever they camped.

The Iroquois used the freshly crushed rhizome as a poultice to prevent blood poisoning from bruises. The Chippewa applied the pounded root on plantain leaf to treat scrofulous sores.

The Montagnais used the flower as a poultice for pain. The Eastern Cree called the plant **WA DUSK SKWAMUK**, and used the root for bruises and burns.

Colonel Lydius, an early explorer wrote. "The Indians take the root, wash it clean, boil it a little, then crush it between a couple of stones. They spread this crushed root as a poultice over leg ulcers. At the same time, the leg is bathed with the water in which the root is boiled. I have seen great cures by the use of this remedy."

The flowers produce a fine blue infusion that serves as a pH test for acid and alkali, turning red upon exposure to acid, or blue when alkaline.

It is hardy to zone three and grows well in wet to moist soils, or shallow water; and prefers some shade.

Early settlers used it as a cathartic, because it looked so much like European iris relatives.

Various native tribes like the Chippewa used blue flag roots as poultice for sores, and swellings. The Cree used it to increase the flow of bile, and as a purgative. The Eastern Mi'kmaq call it "beaver root", due to its preferred place as a home.

The stems were used to make thread, cord and strings for fishing lines, nets, as well as woven baskets and mats.

The Fox knew it as a root to decoct for colds and lung trouble, while the Penobscot steamed the plant throughout their lodges for "disease in general, or chewed the root to kill sickness, and keep disease away."

When I lived in northern Alberta, I planted some *Iris versicolor* near a waterhole. Imagine my surprise, upon my return twenty years later, to see the whole pool surrounded by these beautiful smiling faces!

In the 12th century, King Louis VII of France, while organizing the Second Crusade, had a vision, and named the Siberian iris his "fleur-de-Louis". Other stories suggest he found the iris in Egypt and carried it back to France, and had the fleur-de-lis carved on his coat of arms. Another version suggests it was chosen by the 14th century navigator Flavio Gioja to mark the north point of the compass in honor of the King of Naples, who was of French descent.

Other authors attribute this to *Iris pseudacorus*; and suggest Lys is not a lily but a common flower native to the Lys River in France. Or Lys may be from the Celtic **LI** meaning white.

In Quebec, the fleur-de-lys flies on the provincial flag, and many residents call blue flag, by the same name.

Although the Madonna lily had been the official floral emblem since 1963, in the spring of 2000 this was officially changed.

Iris is the official cultivated flower of Tennessee and Nashville is known as Iris City.

Siberian Iris, despite its name, grows across all of temperature Eurasia, and is hardy to zone 4. It has numerous cultivars, and as the name suggests does well in cold winter climates.

Bearded Iris will rot and die in permanently wet areas. The ideal spot is a sheltered flowerbed against the west or south side of the house, according to Lois Hole, our beloved, former lieutenant-governor of Alberta.

Oregon Iris (*I. tenax/I. gormanni*) grows on the Pacific coast from Washington to Oregon. It is not hardy enough for our winters but is included in the homeopathic section for interest. Grieve says that a tincture of the whole plant, or the bulbous stems is given in bilious vomiting, and is recommended for depression. Natives of the area used the fibres for making rope. In fact, tenax refers to toughness or tenacity of the fibre. Douglas writes "the snare is used in taking elk, and long- and black-tailed deer, and in point of strength it will hold the strongest bullock and is not thicker than the little finger."

Yellow Flag (*I. pseudacorus*) is a native of Great Britain, Ireland, and Europe, but naturalized to this continent, hardy to zone 4, and common in southern BC. It is the hardiest of the water irises, and worthy of a trial.

Its specific name refers to the similarity to *Acorus calamus*, or sweet flag. Pseudo, of course, is from the Greek meaning false. The Romans called it **CONSECRATIX**, because it was used in purification; and Pliny mentions certain ceremonies used in digging it up. Yellow Flag was formerly used in medicine as a powerful cathartic, but because of it extremely acrid nature is no longer used.

Infusions of the rhizome are effective in stopping diarrhea, and it is reputed to have some value in dysmenorrhea and leucorrhea, according to Grieve.

Gerard recommended it for cosmetics. "The root, boiled soft, with a few drops of rosewater upon it, laid plaisterwise upon the face of man or woman, doth in two daies at the most take away the blackness and blewnesse of any stroke or bruise."

He recommended "an oil made of the roots and flower of the Iris, made in the same way as oil of roses and lilies. It is used to rub in the sinews and joints to strengthen them, and is good for cramp." Older authorities praised it for curing toothache, a slice of the fresh rhizome rubbed against the aching tooth.

Culpepper believed the distilled water of the whole herb good for weak eyes, and an ointment of the flowers very good for ulcers or swellings.

A French chemist, in the early 1800s discovered the seeds, when ripe, produce a beverage similar to coffee, and even superior in flavour, after careful roasting. The flowers produce a beautiful yellow dye, and the roots a black dye or ink, when mordant is iron.

Recent work, during a survey of natural fungitoxins, found the leaves of *I. pseudacorus* when stressed with cupric chloride, produce flavonoids and isoflavonoids of commercial interest.

Florentine Iris (*I. germanica* ssp. *florentina*) is called orris root. It has scented white flowers with a bluish flush and yellow beard.

The ancient coat of arms of Florence, a white Iris on a red shield, seems to indicate the city was famed for the growing of these beautiful plants. Many botanists now believe that Florentine is a variety of *I. germanica* with white flowers. It is hardy to zone 2b.

German Iris was used, by 14th-15th century manuscript copiers, to produce green ink. The juice of the blue flowers is purple when pressed and when alum is added a beautiful, clear green is formed.

It is cultivated extensively in Italy for its roots that are prized in perfumery after drying for at least three years. The first use of orris in perfumery dates back to Dominican priests operating a factory in Florence in the early 1600s. Today, only about 170 acres are cultivated. This long drying period has been necessary, in the past, to allow the irone content to develop.

A technique by Ehret and Lerch, *Hort Science* 1998 33:6 has shortened this maturation to a few days. A strain of bacteria, *Rahnella aquatilis*, can synthesize irones from precursors in the rhizomes within one week. Could this work on other species?

The ancient Greek and Romans used florentine iris extensively in perfumes; while Macedonia, Elis, and Corinth were famous for their unguents of iris.

One type of Iris was known as **MACHAIRONION**. The rhizome was ground with flour to created a variety of pasta, today known as Macaroni.

Dioscorides held the root in high esteem. The juice was used for cosmetic purposes, and the bruised root in wine was used for dropsy, bronchitis, coughs, hoarseness, chronic diarrhea and congested headaches.

"All of them haue a warming, extenuating facultie, fitting against coughs, and extenuating grosse humors hard to get up…But dranck with wine, they bring out the menses, yea, & the decoction of them is fitting for woman's fomentations which doe mollify & open the places, & for the sciatica being taken by way of infusion, & for Fistulas, & all hollow sores, which it fill up with flesh."

In Germany, orris root was hung in beer barrels as a preservative, and in France in wine barrels to add subtle flavor.

The Japanese prized orris root as a face powder into the 20th century. In medieval times, the iris was grown on thatched rooftops, hence known as Japanese roof iris. This was done deliberately as a source of face powder, as the Emperor had forbidden anything except food crops on the land.

Orris root still holds a spot in the *British Herbal Pharmacopoeia*, and is used for catarrh, coughs, and diarrhea in children. Although listed zone 5 hardy, Lyndon Penner from Martensville, Saskatchewan (2b) writes that he has grown this iris in full sun for four years. I believe with snow cover it will grow in most zone 3 areas.

Dalmatian Iris is a bearded iris from Croatia that has fragrant pale blue-purple flowers with yellow beards, and considered hardy to zone 5. It is often grown as a source of orris. In Russia, the root was used to make a tonic drink with honey and ginger.

The aged root is powdered and used to scent dentifrices, toothpowders, body powders, dry shampoos, and as a fixative for potpourri. The powder was formerly used as a snuff, for the deliberate purpose of sneezing to relieve cases of congested headaches.

Pieces of the dry root can be placed in the mouth and used as a breath freshener.

Orris root, mixed with anise, was used as a perfume for linens as far back as 1480 AD.

Long pieces of the root were formerly shaped, and used for teething babies; or carved into fragrant rosary beads.

Iris tenax, found west of the Cascade Mountains, was used, by early herbalists to treat vomiting and depression.

Wild Iris (*I. setosa*) is found in northern British Columbia, and up into Alaska. It is grown in Japan for its edible rhizome, and known as **HIOGI AYAME.**

Yellow Water Iris (*I. pseudacorus*) flowers, leaves and roots all exhibit activity against gram-negative bacteria.

The rhizome was traditionally used as a powerful cathartic, for diarrhea, coughs, period pain, dropsy, convulsions, and swellings, the latter in form of poultice with water and butter in parts of Scotland.

A Gaelic manuscript of the 15th century said of this iris:

"The plant is hot and dry in the second degree. If its root is gathered in the end of spring it preserves its virtue for two years. It has a laxative, diuretic value, and removes the obstructions of the spleen, the kidneys and the bladder. It is a powerful remedy against troubles of the spiritual organs, and stomach ailments that proceed from flatulence. Its powder put on sores checks proud flesh and cleans them."

The plant is fully hardy, as I have seen it growing at the Botanic Garden in Calgary.

The leaves give a bright green dye and the rhizomes dark blue, grey and black, previously used in the Harris Tweed industry.

The seeds are roasted as a coffee substitute, and the roots dried and powdered as snuff.

North China Iris (*I. pallasii*) is prized in Traditional Chinese Medicine for its seed. Known as **MA LIN TZU**, the seed is dried and used for a variety of conditions. It is hardy to the prairies. A related Iris is used in India to treat obesity.

Douglas Iris, from the coast of California, is not hardy to our zone. The fruit, stem and roots have all tested positive for juvenile hormone activity with *Oncopeltus fasciatus*.

The key to successful transplant of the rhizome is to do it immediately after flowering.

Blue Flag, and other irises, are attacked by the night-flying Iris borer moth (*Macronoctua onusta*) that lays up to one thousand eggs on the dried leaves. Commercially available nematodes can be used that enter the borer and release a bacterium that kills the caterpillar, and the nematodes then finish up the meal.

MEDICINAL

CONSTITUENTS- *Iris versicolor*- root- phenolic glycosides, iridin, myristin, iriversical (active ingredient), isophthalic acid, (6R, 10S, 11S)-26&17-hydroxyiridal; 17,26-dihydroxyiridal; 10-deoxy-17-hydroxyiridal; iron, copper, cobalt, and oleoresin; salicylic acid, lauric acid, isophthalic acid 0.002%, stearic acid, palmitic acid, I-triacontanol, beta sitosterol, starch, gums, tannins, sterols and furfural, a volatile oil.

I. missouriensis- missouriensin (6 alpha-acetyl-21 beta hydroxyl-hop-22(29)-ene; missourin (6 6 alpha-hydroxy-A'-neogermmacer-22(29)-en-30-oic acid; 7 beta hydroxystigmasterol; 7 beta-hydroxy sitosterol; two novel quinones, irisoquin and deoxyirisoquin; missourin, a novel triterpene; and two cytotoxic triterpenes zeorin and isoiridogermanol; irisoquin, betulinic acid, 7-oxositosterol; irisones A and B; 5,7-dihydroxy-2',6-dimethoxy iso-flavone; 7-oxostigmasterol; mangiferin; 7 beta-hydroxy stigmasterol and sitosterol.

seed- irisquinone (49%), various benzoquinones, hydroquinones and phenols.

I. florentina and *I. germanica* roots- irones, particularly alpha, beta and gamma irones, triterpenes iridal, and irigermanal; beta sitosterol, flavonoids and isoflavonoids including irilon, iriflogenin, irisolone, irigenine, isoflorentin, irogenin, homotectorin, irofloside, iridin, iriskashmirianin 4'-0-beta-D-glucoside, nigricin 4'-0-beta-D-glucoside, irilone 4'-0-beta-D-glucoside, and tectoridine; xanthones such as C-glycosylxanthones, alpha and beta amyrin, iristectorigenin A, myristic acid, and starch.

The first bicyclic and monocyclic triterpenes in nature were isolated from Iris rhizomes.

I. pallasii seed- fatty oils, starch, irisquinone.

Blue flag rhizome appears to clear many of the symptoms associated with low blood sugar, including tired, faint, and lightheaded if one doesn't eat on time.

With too much sugar, they can get hyper, followed by too much release of insulin and then crash with exhaustion. This may be accompanied by a headache, including migraine type that starts with a blur before the eyes and then nausea.

A peculiarity of this headache is that it occurs while the person is relaxing, after stress, and taking a day off. The so-called Sunday headache is perfectly matched to this remedy.

There may be weight on the back of the neck, and a deep depression. They feel that they are carrying the weight of the world on their shoulders.

Blue flag can be very useful in pancreatitis or those suffering flashes of heat after eating sugar or barbecue. The red, glazed complexion of the typical Iris patient looks like sunburn (see face oil below).

I like to use blue flag in cases of lymphatic congestion, where the vessels have become enlarged and congested from obstruction over a long period of time. Ovarian cysts or other pelvic cysts that are boggy and watery respond well to blue flag, combining well with red root. Henry Smith, MD wrote, "Disease in these vessels is a forerunner of chronic skin disease". He is correct.

Blue flag appears to have the ability to increase the rate at which fat is converted into waste. And indeed, cases of psoriasis, eczema, acne, as well as anal fissures related to lymphatic stagnation are helped.

It combines well with yellow dock, burdock root and red clover for many skin problems.

For thyroid deficiencies, or soft goiter that persists for months, try blue flag combined with Oregon grape root. It may help relieve hyperthyroid conditions in some cases, combined with bugleweed and lemon balm of course.

Matthew Wood notes, "it is called for when there are sudden flare-ups of sympathetic excess." Also for mood swings from high to low, according to Australian herbalist Dorothy Hall. One of her students recommended it in menopausal hot flashes.

Matt has seen it work in more than a dozen cases, and characterizes it as a remedy for a "pituitary gone crazy trying to stimulate the ovaries." That is, luteinizing or follicular stimulating hormone is signaling the ovaries and the feedback loop responds no way. The signal becomes more intense and creates chaos.

Noted British herbalist Thomas Bartram uses Blue Flag to restore loss of tonicity to involuntary muscle structures.

A compound called Iridin is used to treat glandular enlargements, especially hypo-function of the stomach. Iridin and Irisin are commercial powdered root extracts with diuretic and intestinal stimulating properties.

Eli Jones used blue flag tincture for tumours of the uterus, as well as spleen enlargement and goiter.

Ellingwood wrote in 1915, that apart from being strongly recommended in psoriasis, "this agent, in from five to ten drop doses every two or three hours, will be found most useful in the treatment of certain cases of eczema of a persistent chronic character, as well as of other pustular and open ulcerating or oozing skin diseases."

One study by Sambhole and Jiddewar, *Sach Ayurvedia* 1985 37:9 found that blue flag given to rats, reduced their food intake. The silly part of the study was a claim that this demonstrates anti-obesity properties.

Another study, by Bambhole, *Ancient Sci Life* 1988 8:117 showed blue flag root significantly increases plasma levels of free fatty acids and glycerol after oral intake. This demonstrates, albeit in an experimental model, the mobilization of fat tissue at 20 mg/kg.

Our local species, *Iris missouriensis*, is actually more powerful than its eastern cousin, according to Michael Moore. The fresh roots are caustic and toxic, but can be poulticed on skin sores, especially effective against staph. The root pulp is wrapped in cotton and applied to the skin rash, repeated as necessary.

The root has a stimulating effect on production of both pancreatic enzymes and bile.

One "00" capsule between meals, or during a three day fast with vegetable or fruit juices is a good way to make dietary changes. One capsule between meals can help in cases of bile insufficiency that manifests as poor oil absorption or light-colored feces.

It was formerly used in treating jaundice, as its bile stimulating effect causes a reflex stimulation of some liver functions.

However, it should not be used for chronic or acute liver malfunction. It does combine well with red root and echinacea for stimulating the lymphatic function.

Small, frequent doses of Blue Flag are a strong diuretic that can help dropsy. It will stimulate saliva and sweat, suggestive of its strong parasympathetic nervous system influence, according to Michael Moore. It should be used in combination with less energetic plants forming the majority of the formula.

The bruised leaves in water are reported to help clear leucorrhea that is white and fluid.

Three components of *I. missourensis*, have been shown to possess cytotoxic activity against P-388 cells. Zeorin has an ED50 of 1.1 micrograms/mL; iso-iridogermanal 0.1 mcg/mL, and missourin, 8.5 mcg/mL. Irigenin has been found to stimulate RNA synthesis. Betulinic acid, also present in birch, shows anti-inflammatory, and tumour preventative activity.

The root of *I. germanica* contains a number of isoflavonoids with anti-inflammatory activity. Rahman et al, *J Ethnopharmacology* 2003 86:2-3.

The triterpenoid iridals show activity against the human tumour cell lines A2780 and K562, as well as anti-plasmodial activity similar to other plants taken as malarial phyto-medicine. The iridals showed cytotoxicity with an IC50 in the 0.1-5.3 mcg/ml range, with some more effective than doxorubicine. Bonfils et al, *Planta Medica* 2001 67:1 and *Phytochem* 2003 62:5.

Work in Japan, looked at methanol and water extracts of 59 plants for anti-ulcer activity.

The root of *I. germanica* was found to possess potent activity from methanol extraction. Muto et al, *Yakugaku Zasshi* 1994 114:12.

Ethanol extracts of the rhizome show significant lowering of cholesterol and triglyceride levels in rat studies. Choudhary et al, *J Ethnopharm 2005* 98:1-2.

Iristectorigenin A, from the root, has been found to exhibit hypotensive activity and inhibit DOPA decarboxylase. The isoflavone, irigenin inhibits cAMP phosphodiesterase.

Myristic acid, most commonly found in nutmeg, is present in *I. florentina* rhizomes.

Its esters are used for perfume and flavouring, as well as shaving cream, lubricating soaps and to waterproof leather.

The seed of North China Iris, or **MA LIN TZU** is used in Traditional Chinese Medicine, for its action on the spleen and lung meridians. The seed in decoction is given to clear up heat, remove dampness, control bleeding and remove toxins, in cases of jaundice, dysentery, hemoptysis, epistaxis, cancer, functional bleeding, leucorrhea, pharyngitis and carbuncles.

In laboratory experiments with mice, an ethanol extract of the seeds, especially the surface layer, shows contraceptive effect.

Recently, isoquinone was isolated from the seeds and in mice showed activity against lymph gland tumours, cervix carcinoma, mouse U-14 cancer, hepatoma, lymphatic sarcoma and Erhlich carcinoma.

This is not to say that all iris compounds are health promoting. A triterpenoid isolated from the rhizomes of *I. tectorum* has been found to promote tumour growth. But then again, isolated compounds from carrot root also show that same result.

Iridal-type ompounds from the root show neuro-protective activity. Zhang CL et al, *J Nat Prod* 2014 77(2).

HOMEOPATHY

The main indications for blue flag are headaches that occur mostly on the right side, and are associated with non-working days, especially Sundays.

There may be sour, vinegary vomiting.

Also typical of Iris are the frequently changing pains, which are cutting pains of short duration, mainly on the right side, such as sciatica and neuralgic pain.

On the skin, *Iris versicolor* can have beneficial effect on vesicles and pustules on the head, face, trunk and limbs, with a tendency to suppurate.

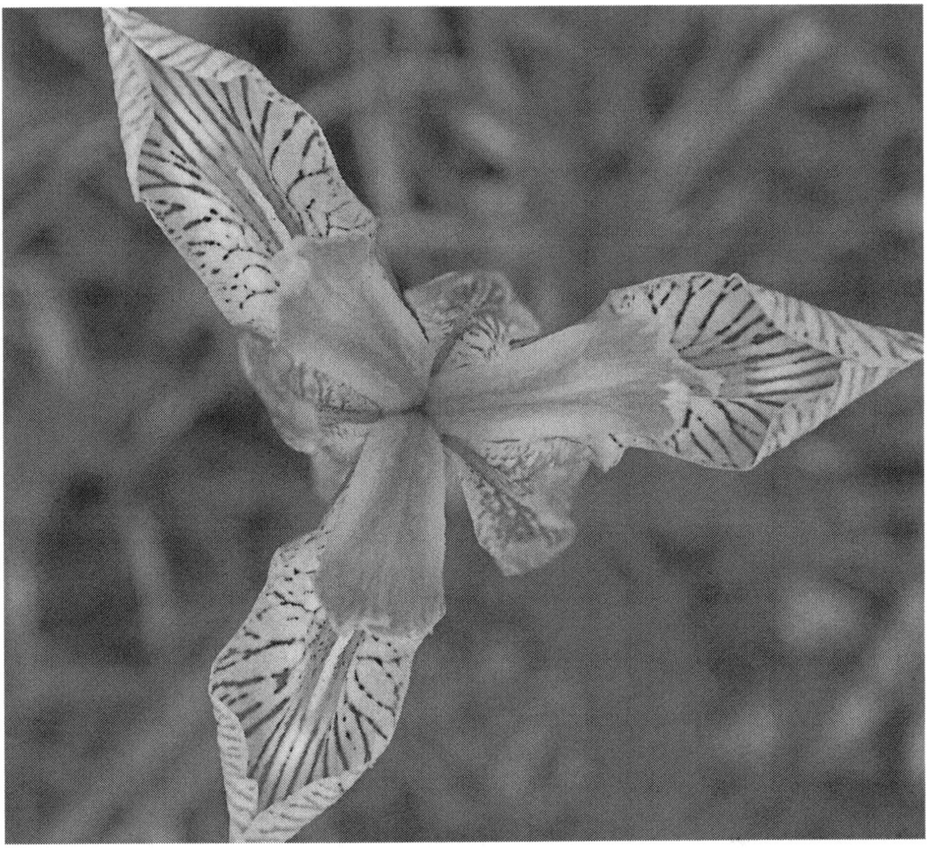

Western Blue Flag

There may be a generalized non-specific depression, and an associated addictive personality attached to this remedy.

There may be anal prolapse often occurring in intestinal colic with a violent urge for stool, frequent passing of watery, mucous stools and burning pains in the rectum, with possible blood.

Should the catarrhal symptoms spread to the renal pelvis, ureter and urethra, the urine will usually have a peculiar, penetrating odour.

It can be used for increasing the flow of bile, and treating goiter of the thyroid.

In Germany, *Iris versicolor* is specific for migraine, facial neuralgia, sciatic neuralgia and conditions following shingles (herpes zoster); as well as inflammation of the gastric mucosa and pancreas.

The Scottish homeopath Douglas Borland typified this individual as "artistic, thin, delicate and nervous; usually very charming people to meet."

DOSE- Tincture to 30th potency. The mother tincture is made from the dry rootstock of the plant, the further north growing the better. Use four ounces of dry root to one pint of 80% alcohol, and let stand for 14 days. Proving by Rowland with four people at tincture, 1st and 3rd dilutions in 1852. Self-experimentation by Burt with green rhizome in 1865, Holcombe with strong tincture in 1867, proving by Wesselhoeft with three females and five males with tincture, 1x, 3x, and 5x in 1867, proving by Berridge with one male and one female at 6c in 1869 and proving by Vakil & Vakil with ten provers at 3c in 1988.

Irisinum patients are very restless at night, dreaming of fighting, snakes, digging up corpses and falling into grave. There is a great desire to sleep in daytime. Scalp tight and constricted, back teeth, upper and lower molars feel elongated and sore.

Pain in umbilical region with electrical shocks to epigastric region. Mushy stools, hands hot and dry all night and day.

DOSE-First potency. Self-experimentation by Burt with crude drug and 1x potency in 1866. This is based on the crude oleoresin of iridin, extracted and promoted by King and other Eclectics of the day.

Bearded or German Iris (*I. germanica*) is related to above, but is used primarily for dropsy and freckles.

DOSE- see above.

Oregon Iris (*I. tenax*) is the remedy for dry mouth, with a deathly sensation at point of stomach. It is for pains of the ileo-caecal region, and recommended in cases of appendicitis.

It is also used for helping ease the pain of adhesions after surgery.

Great exhaustion, burning in mouth and throat. Strange sensation in her mind, thought some of her friends had died. The impression was so strong that she sat down and had a good cry (after 6th dose of 2x).

DOSE- see above. Original proving by Wigg, and his wife, with strong tincture and 2x dilution in 1885.

Iris tenax 30c has had a long clinical reputation of being effective with an attack of appendicitis...Dr. Jacques Imberechts has found it effective in dealing with scar tissue in the right iliac fossa and this I have confirmed...Give also for tenderness of McBurney's point, frequency according to severity. **FOUBISTER**

McBurney's point is between four and five centimeters superomedial to the anterior superior spine of the ilium, on a straight line joining the process and the umbilicus, where pressure elicits tenderness in acute appendicitis.

ESSENTIAL OIL

CONSTITUENTS- *I. germanica* "florentina"- 58-66% cis alpha irone, 34-39% cis gamma irone from Moroccan orris butter.
I. pallida "Dalmatica"- 26-41% cis alpha irone and 55-69% cis gamma irone.

The root of blue flag has been steam distilled when dry and yields 0.025% of a yellow, somewhat unpleasant odour. It has a specific gravity of 0.9410, and contains furfurol, the only constituent able to be identified.

An essential oil is obtained from the pulverized dried roots of either *Iris pallida*, or *Iris germanica ssp. florentina.* A wax-like butter is obtained (often incorrectly called a concrete), that is then washed with alcohol to obtain an absolute. Sometimes an orris resinoid or true concrete are available commercially.

The roots are peeled, washed, dried and pulverized, after at least three years storage, or no scent develops. When fresh, the rhizomes smell somewhat like fresh cut potatoes.

Research in Italy shows that drying the rhizomes, unpeeled, saves 17% of production and also reduces costs.

The oil solidifies at room temperature to a cream-coloured mass with a woody, violet scent and soft floral, fruity undertone. For this reason it is often called Orris butter, or *Beurre d'Iris*. It is produced by steam distillation of *I. pallida* and other irises.

The oil is composed mainly of myristic acid (83-96%), a stearin-like substance that is odour-less but gives the oil solidity. It contains sesquiterpenes like gamma ionone, acetovanillone (0.5%), esters including ethyl myristate; aldehydes like furfural as well as alpha and beta benzaldehydes.

The distillation of orris rhizomes demands a lot of experience and involves a few problems. The yields are low, there is a high amount of starch in the roots, and the volume of pulverized materials, all create headaches for the distiller. It melts at body temperature, and hence a butter.

An absolute is produced by alkali washing in ethyl ether solution that helps remove the myristic acid from the "concrete" oil. It is white or pale yellow with a delicate, sweet floral-woody odour. Both the concrete or butter oil and absolute are used in high-class perfumery.

Recent work in Europe has shown that bacterial treatment with *Rahnella aquatilis*, of the fresh rhizomes shortens maturation time from three years to a few days.

In extreme dilutions, the root flavour becomes sweet and fruity, somewhat reminiscent of raspberries. It is occasionally used in trace amounts in raspberry, strawberry and other fruit flavours.

The average use level is only slightly higher than the minimum perceptible concentration of 0.0005-0.0010 mg%. One part of orris absolute is distinctly perceptible in 200 million parts of sweetened water.

It is offered according to its content of alpha irone, commercial lots from 8-15%.

A resin, or resinoid is prepared from simple alcohol extraction of the peeled rhizomes.

The resin is brown or a dark orange viscous mass with a deep woody, sweet and tobacco-like scent that is very tenacious. The resin is used in soaps, colognes and perfumes. In fact, it is a principal ingredient in about 32% of all modern perfumes of quality.

Many flavour houses produce their own Orris aroma or Orris distillate for use in perfumes. It is used in licorice candy such as Sen Sen, where the sweet root-like notes blend well with the licorice extract.

All forms of orris combine well with cedar wood, sandalwood, vetiver, cypress, mimosa, labdanum, bergamot, clary sage, rose, violet and other florals.

Its an expensive oil, and very often adulterated. True orris absolute is about three times the price of jasmine absolute. The essential oil is used in aromatherapy for is anti-catarrhal, expectorant and mucolyctic properties.

It is often used in combination with other oils for chronic bronchitis and asthma; as well as various skin problems and parasites.

Carotenol extracted from the essential oil of carrot seed (13-19%), and cedrol from various Cedars, have analogues with irone, and various ionones that have a marked resemblance to irone.

The fresh rhizome of orris smells like a freshly cut potato, but changes with age.

Iris pallida was mentioned by Gerard, who wrote, "flowers do smell exceeding sweete, much like the orange flower." To others it is more similar to civet or vanilla.

Iris graminea flowers smell of ripe plums, and *I. foetidissima* leaves and roots smell exactly like roast beef. The Yellow Iris (*I. pseudacorus*) rhizome contains a delicate essential oil that was used in the past to adulterate calamus.

FACE OIL

Matthew Wood recommends that those who have the reddened complexion of the Iris constitution use the Weleda Iris soaps, lotions and creams. I couldn't agree more.

Cytobiol™ Iris is a complex based on the astringent effects of *Iris germanica* combined with zinc and vitamin A, for skin health and treating acne.

HYDROSOL

The distilled water of the whole herb, flowers and roots (Yellow Flag), is a sovereign good remedy for watering eyes, both to be dropped into them, and to have cloths or sponges wetted therein, and applied to the forehead. It also helps the spots and blemishes that happen in and about the eyes, or in any other parts. The said water fomented on swellings and hot spreading ulcers of women's breasts, upon cancers also, and those spreading ulcers called Noli me tangere, do much good. **CULPEPPER**

To cause hair to grow. Take water of flower de luce (orris root) and wash thy head therewith, and it shall cause hayre to grow. **GERARD**

FLOWER ESSENCES

Iris (*I. germanica*) flower essence is for inspiration, and artistic creativity. It helps to eliminate the frustrations due to lack of inspiration or a feeling of imperfection. It helps bring creative and artistic inspiration. **DEVA**

Blue Flag (*I. versicolor*) flower essence activates inspiration and creativity, applicable to the arts. The essences magnify properties in the right brain, which is where much artistic inspiration originates. The right brain helps assimilate information arriving from the chakras, which is then released through the left-brain. Some of the art forms influenced are dance, music, painting and sculpture.

Iris helps people crippled such as in wheelchair to adjust to this condition and to release their artistic creativity. **GURUDAS**

Iris (*I. douglasiana*) flower essence is for those lacking inspiration or creativity; feeling weighed down by the ordinariness of the world. It helps inspire artistry, deep soulfulness which is in touch with higher realms. **FLOWER ESSENCE SOCIETY**

Iris (*I. tenax*) flower essence is for starting over into a radical change of lifestyle that initially may creates chaos and discord, but in the long run will serve the greatest good and harmony. It is for strength combined with humility, for tenacity, and never giving up once one has made a choice from one's integrity. **HUMMINGBIRD**

Blue Iris (*I. germanica*) essence is used for unblocking creativity because blue is the color of the throat chakra, the Taurus, or creative center. **JADE MTN**

Blue Flag (*I. missouriensis*) flower essence is for those having a difficulty managing stress and dealing with crises; those "stuck in the bog", and fall back into addictions and old habits, or those fascinated by external and superficial beauty. **LIVING FLOWER**

Purple Iris (*I. germanica*) essence overcomes deep resentment and-just like bad breath or body odor-it's nasty and off-putting to other. But in my mind, with Purple Iris "stinking thinking" turns into "happy chappy". **OLIVE**

Yellow Flag (*I. pseudacorus*) flower essence is for when the solar plexus is out of balance, for low energy, and to promote change on all levels. **BRYNAHERB**

SPIRITUAL PROPERTIES

The signature for hypoglycemia is seen in the quickly wilting sensitivity of the flower. Iris will shine forth with it beauty one moment, but the next it wilts and fades away. This reminds us of the hypoglycemic person, who fades so easily because of sugar sensitivity.

In Chinese Medicine, the "organ" to which Iris would correspond is the "Triple Burner". This organ is conceived of as three burning cavities in which the fire of the body regulates the water and the water regulates the fire.

Hypoglycemic symptoms would be referred to the Triple Burner because sugar is a major fuel for metabolism (burning) in the body. The seedpod of the Iris consists of three partitions, perfectly depicting the Triple Burner.

This plant grows in excess water and its own Triple Burner has to be emphasized in order for it to survive. **WOOD**

Like the rainbow, the beloved iris (*I. germanica*) combines the natural forces of water and light in an unusually powerful way. It can adapt to extreme dryness or moisture because its rhizomes, stalks, and leaves have special layers that protect them.

The top of each new leaf looks as though it were covered with dew, but these droplets come from inside the plant, secreted through special cracks, giving its leaf its own moist micro-climate, keeping it smooth and soft.

Interestingly, the ability to retain water makes iris a homeopathic remedy for migraine, the head pain caused by pressure of excessive fluid in the brain's blood vessels. **MURPHY**

Its three petals ever reaching upwards toward heaven represent the Trinity, Father, Son and the Holy Ghost. They also speak of the trinity of man, body, soul and spirit, reaching upwards in supplication for guidance. Three petals turn earthward, representing our daily lives, each having a sprinkling of gold, symbolic of deity or God's presence with us every day. With the three upward petals there is another set of three pushing upward in the style crests. These four sets of three symbolize the twelve disciples chosen by Christ.

TRI-STATE IRIS SOCIETY

Orris root is considered a moon herb, so it is useful in digging deep into the subconscious and uprooting what is hidden there. Place it near your journal or hold it while you are meditating to uncover the causes of unresolved issues. **GREGG**

Like the goddess she is named for, Iris teaches us to value the dark murky "lower world" aspects of human experience and to trust the processes that pull us into inner worlds. **DEB FRANCES ND**

PERSONALITY TRAITS

Women require Iris more commonly than men. Sometimes the Iris type will be a tall, slender woman with a long, elegant neck, analogous to the plant, which has, as it were, a long, slender neck shooting up from the bog. But not all Iris subjects need be women or slender. Another group are "pleasantly plump and occasionally fat. They have a weight problem which is often related to addictive food-cravings.

Another strong constitutional trait is that the skin has a "sugary red glaze". A strong emotional trait is attraction to sumptuous people, foods, and objects, which are addictive.

She is exhausted, feels as if there were a weight on her neck, bearing her down to the ground. **WOOD**

Blue Flag presents a picture of emotional ups and downs, hormonal imbalances, glandular disorders and even hysterical outbursts of an irrational kind.

They are a puzzle to themselves, let alone to the struggling diagnostician. Many of these patients try very hard indeed to clear up their own health, to control emotional sensitivity and to eat right and think positive- often to no avail.

What is needed is a deep-seated re-balancing and readjustment of glandular function, especially that of the adrenal glands, the thyroid and that most difficult gland to balance, the pancreas.

The long term Blue flag picture is one of waste removal become inefficient because the body's regulating systems have slipped right off the balance arm altogether.

Without good hormone production, secretion and control, the body is a wildly erratic organism where even great willpower and loads of positive thinking will slide off ineffectively.

All endocrine and lymphatic glands are stimulated to better secretion and discharge of their hormones into bloodstream and tissue fluids by this herb.

The positive Blue Flag from birth, with endocrine harmony and active lymph flow, is a child of clear genetic background. There will be a family history of simple living, good food grown at home, strong physical energy output and healthy old age. We should all be so lucky!
HALL

The iris flower that raises its lovely blooms high above the mud in which it grows is symbolic of the iris personality. Physically, iris people may be tall and slender, attractive, even beautiful, and may give the impression of being delicate. Artistic and charming, they are good at hiding their own insecurities and unhappiness.

They may in fact be depressives, struggling with addictions and abusive relationships and having troubling dreams of corpses and graves.

The flower hold up its head to the heavens, but the person feels a weight upon his neck that bows him down as though he is overburdened. **CLARE GOODRICK-CLARKE**

The keynote symptom I have found most valuable is 'feeling as if stuck in the mud, as if there was a weight on the neck.' **WOOD**

DOCTRINE OF SIGNATURES

The three layers of the flower correspond to the three levels of the psyche, known as the higher, conscious and lower self. Iris represents our choice to be stuck in the "lower self" of addictions and unawareness.

The rootstalks have the ability to store water and feed it to the plant as needed. This is indicative of learning to pace ourselves, building stamina and not burning all our energy up at once.

The simplicity, beauty, and grace of the flower is indicative of its inherent nature and its ability to rise from the bog, reach toward the sky, and honor its beauty.

Matthew Wood observes, "This 'hibernation' is her period of testing. Will she get stuck and return to the bog from which she is attempting to rise, or will she shoot up and show that it is towards heaven that she looks?" **PALLASDOWNEY**

ASTROLOGY

The liver is ruled by Jupiter, the planet of expansion and acquisitiveness. The Jupiter individual may be covetous and consume with the eyes, wanting more than he needs, whether possessions or food or experiences. These individuals exhibit a desire to collect the world, like the tourist who snaps a picture of a famous monument and then rushes on to the next, not taking the time to enjoy the actual experience of beauty…the desire is really for spiritual growth, but, just as the iris is literally "bogged down," he may be tethered to materialism—that is, the person will go on acquiring material possessions. Unable to live themselves, there may be an element of self-disgust, and they may be unable to laugh at themselves.

Worried, troubled, anxious, they need to take the wider view. In the negative state, a troubled liver, low spirits, despondency, and low stamina are all typical of those needing this remedy. Taken over time, the face will become clear and the eyes more radiant as the individual begins to realize his true spiritual self. **GOODRICK-CLARKE**

RECIPES

TINCTURE- 5-10 drops 3x daily. Too much can be cathartic and unpleasant. The dry root only tincture should be made in early spring or in fall after tops have died down. Use a 1:5 ratio of 80% alcohol. For tumours of the uterus, use 25 drops three times daily. Tinctures from orris root for perfume work are produced with 95% alcohol.

BLUE FLAG LEAF- Bruise the juice from leaves in one half-cup water. Use 10-20 drops three times daily in a retention douche for leucorrhea.

CAPSULES- Two "00" of the ground dried root powder.

DECOCTION- One half teaspoon of dried root simmered in pint of water for ten minutes.

IRIS SEED- 3-9 grams.

GYPSY REMEDY FOR COUGHS- Combine one part orris root with two parts ivy. Cover with 75% alcohol for four weeks. Use 10 drops as needed in some water with honey.

DENTIFRICE- Combine equal parts of orris root powder and baking soda.

Note: The active principles are not very water soluble, so tinctures are preferred.

CAUTION- Do not use during pregnancy or lactation. It is too strong for children. Use Blue flag for short periods of time, and never in deficient conditions. Use only dry root.

Blue Flag is contraindicated with acute liver, pancreatic or GI disease, and in cases of cholecystitis.

BOGBEAN
BUCKBEAN
(*Menyanthes trifolium*)
(*M. trifoliata* L.)
PARTS USED- leaves, rhizomes

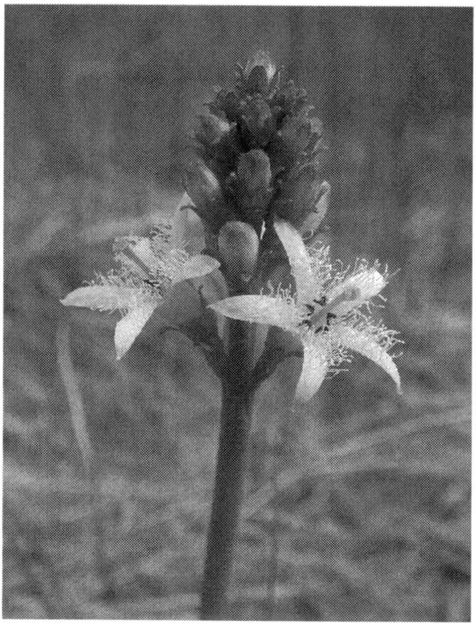

Bogbean flower

Buckee, Buckee, biddy Bene
Is the way now fair and clean?
Is the goose y gone to nest?
And the fox y gone to rest?
Shall I come away?
OLD NURSERY RHYME

Menyanthes may be from the Greek **MENANTHOS** for moon or month flower; due to life of the flowers or related to the lunar cycle. Or its name came from Theophrastus, a Greek botanist, **MENYEIN** for disclosing, and **ANTHOS** flower, in allusion to the sequential opening of flowers. Other authors believe Menyanthes is derived from the Greek **MINUTHO**, to diminish, for the short-lived flowers.

Buckbean is from the Dutch **BOKSBOON** or French **BOUC** for Goat's Bean. Bogbean has similar foliage to broad beans. It should be noted that **SHARBOCK** the German for scurvy is also considered a possible origin of the word.

It is abundant, but easily passed by in mosquito infested bogs and swamps it inhabits. The delicate whitish-pink flowers give off a very unpleasant odor when in bloom.

Alaska natives use the rhizomes as an emergency food supply, just as Laplanders made bread from the powdered root. Flours from buckbean can be substituted for wheat and other grains that may cause allergies, where the plant is plentiful.

Early herbals list the leaf as a hop substitute in beer; one Swedish recipe from 1824 suggesting one part buckbean for every eight parts hops. Today, the bitter principles are used in liqueurs.

The leaves are best collected in flower, but since they produce for three months, this is not really a problem. The root can be collected but should not be over-harvested.

Native tribes of this region made decoctions of the stem and root for stomach sickness; especially if there was spitting of blood. Other tribes drank the tea to put on weight lost during the flu. The Kwakiutl of BC decocted and drank the root water for stomach troubles. In Scotland, stomach ulcers were likewise treated.

For constipation, the root is boiled until the water is thick and dark. One teaspoon at a time is given.

Buckbean leaves make an effective facial steam for acne, or suitable rinse for oily hair.

The dried leaves are a common smoking ingredient, blending well with mullein, clover, coltsfoot, bearberry and other fragrant herbs.

Johannes Franckenius in 1613 noted bogbean decoctions remove all visceral obstructions, act as emmenogogues, diuretics, kill intestinal worms, and were an efficacious remedy in scrofula. Seed decoctions were used for rheumatism.

Cullen suggested using the root for obstinate skin affections of a cancerous nature; applied externally in the form of a fresh poultice.

Boerhaave cured his gout by drinking the plant juice in whey.

Studies from the former USSR indicate that bogbean successfully removes mercaptan compounds from pulp and paper wastewaters.

Buckbean contains mitsugashiwa lactone that induces the catnip response in cats.

It was believed that drinking buckbean herbal tea every day makes you live longer. Who's to say?

MEDICINAL

CONSTITUENTS- aerial parts- numerous anthraquinones including emodin, aloe-emodin, chrysophanol, menyanthin, and secologanin, menthiafolin and dihydro-foliamenthin glycosides, sweroside, choline, tannins 3%, physcion, menthiafolin, franula-emodin, rham-nicoside, seco-iridoid and alaterin. Alkaloids like gentianin E, gentianadine, gentiatibetine and gentianlutine. Various phenolics such as ferulic and caffeic acids, p-hydroxybenzoic and protocahtechuic acids.

Fats such as palmitic acid, phytosterin and ceryl alcohol, as well as flavonoids such as rutin, hyperoside, trifolin; pigment like carotin; enzymes such as invertin and emulsin; a terpenoid lactone loliolide, various triterpene glycosides such as lupeol, betulin, betulinic acid, and beta amyrenol, coumarins like scopoletin, scoparone and braylin; as well as mitsugashiwa lactone.
Root- betulinic acid 0.8%. betulin, loganin, foliamenthin, sucrose, loganetin, pentosans, pectin, meliatin, inulin, alpha spinasterol, alpha and beta lupeol were identified.

Bogbean is very useful in conditions where digestion and blood quality are involved. The herb is cooling, cleansing and detoxifying. Because its chief action is to clear old stagnation, it is similar to gentian root, stimulating the vagus nerve and increasing sympathetic nervous system activity.

It is useful for pitta/kapha tendencies in the Ayurvedic tradition, and for damp heat and liver Qi stagnation from TCM.

Swedish studies confirm decoctions of buckbean show inhibition of inflammatory models *in vivo*, and *in vitro*. Huang et al, *Yao Hsueh Hsueh Pao* 1995 30.

This makes it useful in difficult conditions like fibromyalgia; combining well with black cohosh.

Bogbean stimulates sympathetic deficient and sedates excessive parasympathetic nervous systems. It is worth a trial in cases of anorexia, combining well with calamus root. It works well for amenorrhea in women with vacuity of the blood or the spleen, and hence the older German name **MONATSBLUME**, or Moonflower.

Bogbean's bitter principles relieve spleen, liver and intestinal obstruction. Deocyloganin, for example, possesses laxative properties.

As a bitter digestive stimulant, it promotes appetite, taken in cold water ten minutes before meals. This makes it useful for frontal headaches associated with eating fatty foods, and indigestion or constipation associated with biliousness and bloating.

The bitter index of Bogbean is 2.5-3 times less than Gentian at one part to 4-10 million. Caffeic and ferulic acid are bile stimulants.

Sweroside and loganin are constituents that give this plant strong hepatoprotection. Luo et al, *Chem Pharm Bull* (Tokyo) 2009 57:1.

As a diaphoretic, taken in hot water, it is used for treating intermittent fevers and acute viral infections. The German name **FIEBERKLEE** means Fever Clover, indicating a long usage for remittent or intermittent fevers.

The lymphatic glands begin to drain, and with its diuretic action, bogbean is well-suited to help many chronic arthritic and rheumatic conditions which find their origin in poor fat and protein digestion.

The fresh juice of the leaves is specific for gouty rheumatism.

Because it detoxifies pelvic lymphatic congestion, buckbean is often helpful in uterine disorders, migraines of liver origin, menstrual irregularities and hemorrhoids. Individuals with allergy or food sensitivities, associated with constipation and indigestion may benefit. In some ways, it is similar to blue flag in the treatment of biliary migraines, but is much less purgative in nature.

Studies out of Lithuania in 1989 suggest that buckbean be further studied for possible anti-tumour activity. Water and alcohol extracts show the plant exhibiting activity against gram-positive bacteria, particularly *Staphylococcus aureus*.

Buckbean relieves wheezing and asthmatic congestion by stimulating expectoration.

Skin problems that stem from stagnation, such as dry flaky skin, eczema, and psoriasis respond to buckbean combined with goldthread, burdock root or Oregon grape root.

Externally, a poultice of buckbean leaves can help soothe festering skin sores, herpes pain, and reduce glandular swelling. A patented shampoo on the market contains buckbean leaf extract for its anti-bacterial properties.

Buckbean combines well with baneberry root externally to relieve achy joints, including osteoarthritis. Gentianine, a leaf alkaloid, shows pain killing and tranquilizing effect.

Gentianadine reduces blood pressure and decreases inflammation. Dr. Bastyr used buckbean leaf tincture, 15 drops three times daily, for hypertension.

Buckbean has been noted to demonstrate hemolytic activity and may increase risk of bleeding in those taking warfarin or similar blood thinners.

Remember, buckbean leaf is for chronic conditions and will severely irritate colitis, or acute diarrhea conditions. In the Highlands of Scotland, the herb is used for stomach pains, including ulcers, but caution is advised.

Aperient, tonic candies are marketed in Europe for infants that contain 0.25% menyanthins, derived from bog bean.

In Japan, the herb is known as **SUISAIYO**, or **MEISAI**. In early herbals, the intake of the plant was said to induce drowsiness, a quality after which it is named.

Although its main traditional use is to strengthen the stomach, it is used for insomnia, indigestion, intermittent fevers, headaches, earaches, amenorrhea, jaundice, edema, gout, scabies and ulcerated furuncles.

The leaf tea may help shingles. J. V. Cerney relates the story of a working man who, "had an eruption of painful little blisters along his lower ribs on his right side. They followed in a line along his ribs and became agonizingly painful to the point where he couldn't do his job." He was completely cured using buckbean leaf tea.

Research by Tunon et al, suggests that bog bean root be used for glomerulonephritis (kidney tubule inflammation). Such inflammations often result during unresolved strep infections. The exact mechanism is unknown, but it is thought that platelet activating factors (PAF) and leukotrienes are involved. Tunon, *Phytomedicine* 1995. Or maybe, this is due in part, to elastase inhibition. Ortiz et al, 1987. The roots have been found to possess hemolytic properties, due to an unidentified substance.

Two of eight compounds found in roots show significant inhibition of prostaglandin synthesis, with 2-14 times the potency of aspirin. This makes the root an important analgesic agent, and explains in part, the folkloric use in rheumatism.

The decocted rhizome shows benefit in acute glomerular nephritis. Bohlin et al, *Journal of Ethnopharmacology* 1993 38 2-3.

Betulinic acid and betulin have shown activity against melanoma cancer and HIV-1. Betulinic acid inhibits prostaglandin synthesis with IC50 of 101, and betulin at 119 microM, suggesting anti-inflammatory activity.

Work by Lindholm et al, looked at bogbean for its anti-cancer activity against ten human cancer cell lines. The herb was one of seven with anti-tumour potential out of 100 plants studied. *Journal Biomol Screen* 2002 7:4.

Kuduk-Jaworska et al, *Z Naturoforsch* 59c 5-6 found the plant contains both immune stimulating and suppressing compounds, and high concentrations of selenium.

One polysaccharide from a water extract showed significant anti-inflammatory effect. The herb induces a suppressive type of dendritic cells that reduces the capacity to induce Th1 and stimulate Th17 of allogeneic $CD4^+$ cells.

This suggests use in autoimmune conditions such as rheumatoid arthritis, multiple sclerosis, asthma and irritable bowel disease. Jonsdottir et al, *J Ethnopharm* 136:1. Care should be observed in IBS due to stimulating and possibly, irritating effect.

It is worthy of a trial in anorexia as well, combining well with purple-leaved bunchberry and calamus root.

HOMEOPATHY

Buckbean is a remedy for certain headaches and intermittent fever. There may be a coldness to the abdomen, accompanied by sensations of tension and compression.

The head pain is improved by applying hard hand pressure. The symptoms are made worse by going up stairs; and improved by stooping or sitting.

There may be ravenous hunger, especially for raw meat, but no thirst. The abdomen is distended and full; and exaggerated by nicotine.

The extremities are icy cold; and the patient's legs may jerk and twitch while laying down. A cold fever may be present.

Thoughts come with difficulty, cross, ill-humored and discontented. Anxious, indifferent to amusements. Dreams of animals and dinosaurs.

DOSE- Third to thirtieth potency. The mother tincture is prepared from the whole fresh plant when coming to flower. Use 3X for pressure headaches, fever attacks, disruption of body heat regulation and trigeminal neuralgia.

First proving by Hahnemann with ten males and tincture.

Teste self-experimented as cited in Clarke.

He remarked. "There are few diseases where *Menyanthes* is indicated which could not be cured much better with *Drosera*. This opinion, however, is founded on my own impressions, which I am always willing to distrust."

ROOT OIL

The fresh roots are gathered and washed, and then pulverized and covered with four parts of olive or canola oil. Let sit warm for one week; shaking daily. Use a low temperature crock pot if temperatures are too cold. Stain and use for arthritic/rheumatic pain.

FLOWER ESSENCE

Buckbean flower essence is for helping one maintain calm repose in the midst of activity. There may be mental confusion, lack of humour, and even aversion to any small amusements. **PRAIRIE DEVA**

PERSONALITY TRAITS

Bogbean has a long history of use in rheumatism. The Bogbean person often has pain in the kidney region that may later affect the legs, knees and feet. There may be heat and swelling in the joints, that are improved with movement. Gouty rheumatism is a classic Bogbean!

Sciatica pain becomes worse as the body congests and stagnates with old acids and waste. Water retention is reduced by making the lymphatic system more efficient.

In the negative state, the Bogbean person cannot climb the stairs. Repeated trips to the chiropractor only give temporary relief.
They need to walk to keep the lymphatic moving and the kidneys eliminating. In this state, they crave meat and yet are not thirsty- a sure recipe for kidney damage. Pain-killers simply overload them more resulting in kidney stones, backache, sciatica and muscle pain; even kidney failure.

In the positive state, the Bogbean type is able to start walking- and do exercises like aquacize, bicycling and golf. Even shopping can take on a quality of enjoyment. **PRAIRIE DEVA**

SPIRITUAL PROPERTIES

The Russian name for Bogbean is ***VAHTA***. An old folk legend tells about a girl of that name. When Vahta was little, she would play in the forest with gnomes and listen to their stories about herbs and other plants. But one day her spiteful stepmother, who was a witch, turned her into a mermaid and banished her to life at the bottom of the river.

Vahta spent many lonely months living in the river, but one day she left to play with her forest friends once more. She forgot that she had to return to the river by sundown, and when she finally returned late in the evening, the Queen of the Underwater Kingdom punished her severely. She made Vahta stand guard at the entrances of all rivers and lakes, never to venture into the forest again. Since that time, local people began to notice a plant with a beautiful white and rose flower that looked like a weeping mermaid. The flowers were so brilliant they could be seen even at night and were always a sign that a river, lake or swamp was nearby. **ZEVIN**

The Buckbean stands for change. All the species of buckbean are marsh plants. They serve to decorate the lakes upon which they float. The buckbean stands for change in situation or sentiment. A gentle, painless change in the order of things, natural and inevitable.

GRIMAUD

RECIPES

FRESH PLANT TINCTURE- Up to four mls four times daily. Use a 50% alcohol extract for maximum benefit of a 1:2 fresh plant extract. For dry plant use a 1:5 ratio. For hypertension, 15 drops 3x daily. Collect leaves in late spring, early summer.

POWDERED ROOT OR LEAF- 1-3 grams as a tonic. Small doses tone and larger ones cause drainage. Go slow!

COLD INFUSION- One fluid ounce repeated every 3-4 hours. Prepare by putting one teaspoon of dried leaf in warm water overnight. Combine with mint or pineapple weed if necessary. The fresh plant can cause vomiting in some individuals.

WINE- roots can be infused in wine for treating gouty arthritis.

FRESH JUICE- One tbsp three times daily for gouty rheumatism.

FLUID EXTRACT- Ten to forty drops as needed.

BUCKBEAN ALE- Take five pounds of malted barley and mash in four gallons of water at 150° F for ninety minutes. Take the four gallons (add more boiling water if needed) and add 45 grams of dried bogbean leaf. Boil one hour. Strain and add two pounds of brown sugar, stir to dissolve. Cool to 70 degrees Fahrenheit and pour into fermenter with yeast. Ferment one week or until complete. Siphon into bottles, add 1/2 tsp of sugar and cap. Ready in two weeks.

CAUTION- Bogbean is contra-indicated in diarrhea, dysentery, biliary obstruction and colitis. Avoid while taking anti-coagulants and anti-platelets like warfarin, heparin or aspirin, and during pregnancy.

The seed is contraindicated in spleen qi deficiency with diarrhea, and during breastfeeding, as it may inhibit lactation.

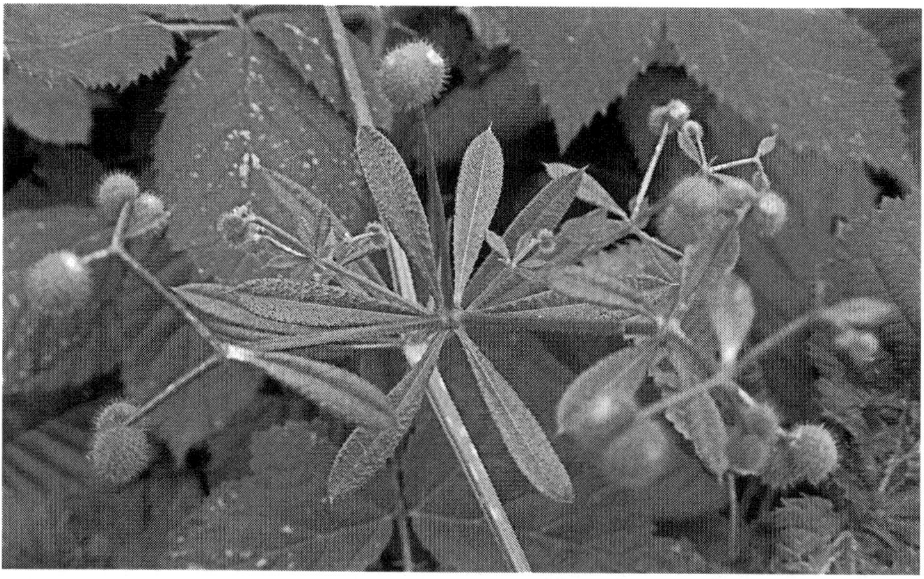

Cleavers

CLEAVERS

(*Galium aparine* L.)

(*G. vaillantii* DC.)

(*G. agreste* Wallr. var. *echinospernum* Waller.)

NORTHERN BEDSTRAW
(*G. boreale* L.)
(*G. septentrionale* Roemer & J.A. Schultes)
(*G. strictum* Torr.)
(*G. hyssopifolium* Hoffm.)
SWEET SCENTED BEDSTRAW
(*G. triflorum* Michx.)
(*G. brachiatum* Pursh)
(*G. circaezans* Michx. var *circaezans*)
YELLOW BEDSTRAW
LADY'S BEDSTRAW
GOOSEGRASS
(*G. verum* L.)
SMALL BEDSTRAW
(*G. trifidum* L.)
FALSE CLEAVERS
(*G. spurium* L.)
SMOOTH BEDSTRAW
WHITE BEDSTRAW
(*G. mollugo* L.)
LABRADOR BEDSTRAW
(*G. labradoricum* [Wiegand] Wiegand)
(*G. tinctorium* L. Scop var. *labradoricum* Weigand)
PARTS USED- leaves, flowers, seeds, roots

Galium is from the Greek **GALA** meaning milk. This may be in reference to the use of cleavers as rennet or milk coagulating substitute, hence the French **GAILLET.** It may be from the Italian **GALA** meaning party. The Greek **GALION** means bedstraw according to one author.

In Scotland, the bedstraw roots were practically depleted from the shiels for the red dye used in Elizabethan party clothes.

These areas became know as gala shiels, and today Galashiels is one of Britain's main clothing manufacture towns.

Aparine is from the Greek **APAIREIN**, meaning to seize, in reference to the tenacious velcro-like hooked stems.

Cleavers is descriptive of how weak stemmed plants depend on others for support, using their hooked bristles to "cleave", meaning to adhere or stick. The term comes from the Old English name for the plant **CLIFE** from Clifian "to stick". In Scotland, it is known as sticky willie, and used as a strainer in making flummery, an oatmeal dish boiled down to jelly.

Goose Grass, Gosling Grass, and Turkey-Grass all allude to feed fit only for farm birds.

Bedstraw comes from the legend that it was part of Jesus' bedding, and hence "our ladies bedstraw".

Galium aparine and *G. verum* are introduced annual and perennial plants respectively; while the others are native perennials, all with similar properties.

Grieve, in her Modern Herbal, suggests that cleavers (*G. aparine*) infusion "has a most soothing effect in cases of insomnia, and induces quiet, restful sleep". Dioscorides considered the plant useful for countering weariness.

The Cowichan rubbed the introduced Cleavers onto their hands to remove tree pitch, the dried plants were tinder for fire.

Northern bedstraw was used, by early settlers, to stuff mattresses and pillows. The Cree use the roots and combine them with high bush cranberries to produce a red dye.

The roots have to be boiled to the correct colour; for too long and it changes to yellow. Known as **KEWETI-NIPEWUSKOSE**, the red dye was used to colour porcupine quills.

Northern, Sweet and Small Bedstraw were all used by the Dena'ina of Alaska as hot packs for aches and pains. They were known as wormwood's partner, or **TS'ELVENI VETS'ELQ'A**.

The sweet scented bedstraw yields a red dye from the roots, while the coumarin rich flowers are used for their exquisite perfume. In Africa, the root extract is combined with *Rumex* species, and taken internally to treat blenorrhagia, a discharge from mucous membranes.

The leaves and flowers of both were infused for diuretic effect; hot packs and foot baths for sore aching muscles.

The young plants make an acceptable potherb, served hot with butter, or cooled and added to salads.

Like yarrow, the plant can be crushed and put in the nose to stop nosebleeds.

Natives of the Pacific Northwest rubbed their scalps with mashed cleavers to stimulate hair growth, and as an astringent facial cleanse.

Fresh infusions of the plant, which taste like oriental green tea, are good for insomnia. Cleavers is related to the coffee family, and the small ripe seeds can be roasted and ground to produce an acceptable beverage with no caffeine. The small, unripe seedheads are useful to lace makers, to pad the top of pins.

Today, the bedstraws are listed as ingredients in underarm deodorants; the cooled tea soothes sunburn, complexion problems and wrinkled skin.

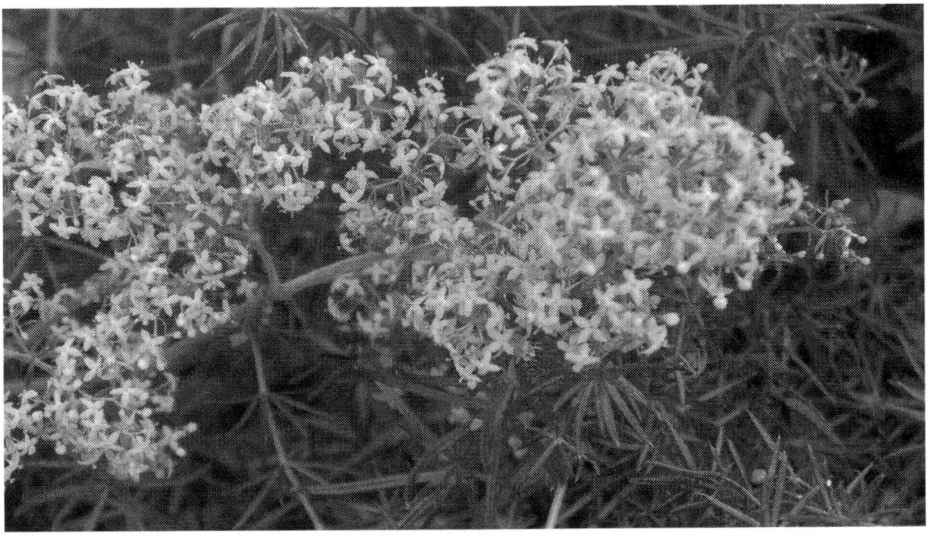

Yellow Bedstraw

The flowers of Yellow Bedstraw (*G. verum*) have a lovely honey fragrance, and were a favourite for stuffing mattresses in Europe in medieval times. It also curdles milk, and gives a yellow colour to the cheese. Early Tuscans used it to make goat and sheep cheese taste sweeter.

Gerard mentions that residents of Namptwich used the plant for rennet "esteeming it to be the best cheese that is made with it, and in some of the Western Isles, they curdle milk with a strong decoction of this herb." The famed Double Gloucester Cheese from England is said to get both its tang and rich colour from the use of yellow bedstraw and stinging nettles as vegetable rennet. The roots give a red dye, made more vibrant, and rich with the addition of stannous chloride as a mordant.

K'Eogh, the Irish herbalist wrote, "when applied to burns, the crushed flowers alleviate inflammation, and when applied to wounds, they can heal them."

Parkinson wrote "these sorts with white flowers have been thought unprofitable, and of no use, but Clausius saith, the poor women in Austria, Hungaria and other places in Germany that gather herbs and roots for their uses that need them, bringing them to the market to sell…by their experience found it good for the sinews arteries and joints, to bath them therewith both to take away their weariness and weakness in them, and to comfort and strengthen them also after travail, cold or pains".

Joseph Miller wrote of Lady's Bedstraw, "some commend a decoction of it for the gout; and a bath made of it is very refreshing to wash the feet of persons tired with over-walking." Native tribes of Eastern Canada used the flowers for light fevers, kidney problems and convulsions.

Small Bedstraw is a native perennial, often mistaken for a shorter Northern Bedstraw. It prefers marshy ground and stream banks throughout the prairies.

The Ojibwa made infusions of the plant for all kinds of skin diseases such as eczema, ringworm and glandular swellings associated with tuberculosis.

Labrador Bedstraw looks similar to *G. triflorum* but is smaller and has four whorls of leaves, instead of the latter's five or six.

False Cleavers is a common introduced annual in gardens and fields. It looks like *G. aparine*, but has greenish yellow flowers, instead of white, and smaller fruits. The plant is very prevalent in Saskatchewan, on deserted fields and old garden plots. Both plants reduce yields of wheat, flax, barley, rape and field peas.

The powdered leaves are used in Africa to treat eczema, and the burnt ash for oral sores.

Smooth or White Bedstraw is an introduced perennial found in Saskatchewan, and in Alberta for the first time in 1994 by Anne Weerstra while walking along the roadside and railway near Jasper. It looks like *G. aparine* but the stems are smooth, not bristly.

Like other members of the genus, it curdles milk, and the root contains high levels of pigments that can be applied to seeds to make them distasteful to birds.

Seedlings of *G. aparine* contain high levels of the anthraquinone aldehyde, nordamnacanthal, which possesses anti-feeding activity against cutworms.

The related *G. aegeum* contains paeoniflorin, also found in Peony root. This is an important medicinal compound.

MEDICINAL

CONSTITUENTS- *G. aparine-* various sterols, iridoids including aucubin, asperulosidic and deacetyl- asperulosidic acids, galiosin, scopoletin, nordamnacanthal, asperul-oside, and monotropein; alkaloids such as protopine, harmine and vasicinone; quinazoline alkaloids (1-hydroxy-deoxypeganine, and 8-hydroxy-2,3-dehydro-deoxypeganine). The whole plant is 11.7% protein, of which 7.3% is digestible. Nitrogen/sulphur ratio is 7:1, with large amounts of zinc (127 ppm).
roots- anthraquinone derivatives, including alizarin, xanthopurpurin and its esters, galiosin and simple anthraquinones, including 2-methyl anthroquinone.
G. boreale- polyphenols (7.7%), galactoside (quercitin) and up to 6% oil.
G. triflorum- coumarin, asperuloside, vanillic acid, and 4-hydroxycinnamic acid.
G. verum- various iridoid monoterpenes including asperuloside, V1, V2, and galioside; monotropein, scandoside, desacetyl-asperulosidic acid, asperulosidic acid, 6-acetylscandoside, giniposidic acid, and daphylloside.
Also contains (+)-pinoresinol, epipinoresinol, (+)-medioresinol, isorhamnetin, diosmetin, diosmetin 7-0-beta-D glucopyranoside, ursolic acid, ursolic aldehyde, rubifolic acid, rennin 1%, various flavonoids including rutin, isorutin, palustroside, cynaroside, anthracene derivatives, and chlorogenic acid. The maximum amount of anthracenes is at start of plant growth in May, and again during flowering in July.
root- alizarin, n-alkanes mainly C29 and C31.

G. spurium- quercitin galactoside, asperulosides, rutin, caffeic, chlorogenic and ursolic acids, saponins
root- alisarin, rubrierythrinic acid, purpurin.
G. mollugo- mollugin, flavonoids, coumarins, phenolic acids, and iridoid glucosides.

Cleavers is used for skin and urinary problems. Skin conditions that are the result of poor lymphatic drainage respond to both internal and external treatment. Dr. Scudder recommended using cleavers for nodulated growths and deposits on the mucous membranes or skin.

King's *American Dispensatory* opens his chapter on cleavers with: "A most valuable refrigerant and diuretic, and will be found very beneficial in many diseases of the urinary organs, as suppression of urine, calculous affections, inflammation of the kidneys and bladder, and in scalding of urine in gonorrhea."

For psoriasis or other dry ulcerative conditions, use fresh infusions for bathing, as well as drinking as a tea. It combines well with calendula, echinacea, nettles and red clover for this purpose. Poultices of the fresh herb and ground oatmeal help reduce tumours, and skin hardened by ganglia.

Cleavers is useful in skin conditions that weep and damp heat skin problems such as psoriasis, combining well with burdock root and yellow dock root.

Inflamed tonsils, adenoids, lumpy breasts, lipomas and other lymphatic inflammation all respond to cleavers. In fact, the salty, bitter flavor helps treat all swollen, hot lymphatic nodes anywhere in body.

Combine with figwort, red root and echinacea for hot painful nodes in neck, armpits and groin. Note that red root is neutral, cleavers is cooling and calendula is warming when used as lymphatic decongestants.

Breasts that are generally fibrous rather than scattered cysts or nodes, may suggest the use of red clover, figwort or Easter lily, according to Matthew Woods.

When taken warm it is useful for the acute fever stage of measles, chicken pox and other childhood viral infections, helping resolve and move to skin surface.

Urinary infections in children, with swollen lymph nodes respond well to cleavers. Eli Jones recommended the use of cleavers for cancer of the tongue, when a nodular growth is noticeable and tender to the touch.

Combine fresh juice with equal parts of vegetable glycerine for skin cancers. It soothes inflamed stretch marks, slow healing burns, and suppurating skin conditions, according to Michael Moore.

Recent work by Thring et al, *BMC Complement Alt Med* 2009 9:27 found cleavers exhibits significant anti-elastase activity. The study found 58% inhibition for the herb, compared to 51% for burdock and 32% for anise and angelica. Rose showed anti-collagenase activity.

It successfully treats kidney and bladder inflammation, scalding urine (including gonorrhea), stone or gravel obstructions, testicular pain and enlarged or inflamed prostate.

For bladder damp heat with dark and difficult urination, combine with amur bark and water plantain root.

Irritability of the vas deferens and seminal vesicles, inflamed prostate and orchitis, or sore testicles, indicate use of this herb.

Cleavers increases circulation of lymph through the dilation of capillaries, at the cellular level, and combined with mild astringency may explain, in part, the healing of gastric ulcers and inflamed urinary tract tissue.

All species contain asperuloside, an anti-inflammatory and mildly laxative agent. This compound and monotropein are about 15 times less stimulating to the bowel than senna, but gentle and effective, nonetheless.

Helen Farmer-Knowles, in her interesting book, *The Healing Garden*, suggests cleavers be used in the treatment of ME (myalgic encephalomyelitis), or chronic fatigue syndrome.

Work in Poland by Gryzbek et al *Int J Pharm* 1997 35 found ethyl acetate extracts of the whole herb displayed moderate anti-viral activity against HIV-1.

Work by Berkowitz et al, *Journal of Organic Chemistry* 1982 47 found asperuloside is chemically converted to prostanoid intermediates.

Cleavers is best thought of as a relaxing, cooling and soothing cleanser. For weight loss, the acids in cleavers speed up the metabolism of stored or adipose fat, combining well with Chickweed, another cooling, heat-clearing herb.

French researchers found extracts of the plant lower blood pressure, as far back as 1947.

During acute hepatitis it helps rid the body of toxins, but without irritating. For this reason, it is useful for alcoholics with fluid retention and urinary symptoms.

It is most powerful as a fresh juice. Applied to slow healing burns, ulcerated skin and inflamed stretch marks, it works very well.

In the East Indies, fresh juice of cleavers has been used to treat gonorrhea. In Portugal, cleavers is used for its diuretic and anti-spasmodic effect in treating kidney problems.

Bedstraw should be considered in formulas treating enlarged thyroid, accompanied by obesity and water retention. Ironically, because of its cooling nature, it should not be used by those who are always cold, and avoided by individuals prone to diabetes.

John Lust recommended cleaver tincture for epileptic seizures too frequent and close together.

The herb combines well with marshmallow for cystitis, with echinacea for throat infections, and with red clover, nettles and figwort for psoriasis.

Matthew Wood has an additional take on cleavers. "It is beneficial in 'gathering of the nerves' and inflammation of the nerve endings, tickling and itchy skin. It is a specific in Dupuytren's contracture and Morton's neuroma, when the tendons tighten up under the middle finger or toes."

In Traditional Chinese Medicine, the plant is used for similar properties and known as **BAAT SIN CHOU** (Mandarin), and **BA XIAN CAO** (Cantonese). I have also seen it called **CHU YANG YAN**.

Peter Holmes adds, "in overall gestalt, Cleavers is close to Japanese Knotweed (Fleece Flower)." Not sure I agree totally.

The plant *G. aparine* var. *tenerum* shows an anti-cancer effect on leukemia.

Galiosin is similar to the dye ingredient in Madder, a close cousin. It has specific anti-inflammatory and spasmolytic effect on the urinary tract and may contribute to the action of breaking urinary stones and staining urine red like Madder.

Yellow Bedstraw is a specific for swollen ankles, as well as a good diuretic for bladder and kidney catarrh. Externally, a poultice or wash of the fresh herb is used for poorly healing wounds, or as a salve for psoriasis.

John Hill noted an infusion will cure the most violent nose bleeds.

It is a bitter tasting herb, with a long reputation in France for treating epilepsy.

Work by Jaric et al, *J Ethnopharm* 111:1 identified sedative activity in this species.

The related *G. verum* var. *leiocarpum* and variety *trachycarpum* are used in TCM, and known as **PENG ZI CAO**.

Sweet Scented Bedstraw (*G. triflorum*) contains blood pressure lowering substances, according to a study conducted by Knott and McCutcheon, *J of Pharmaceutical Sciences* 1961 50:11.

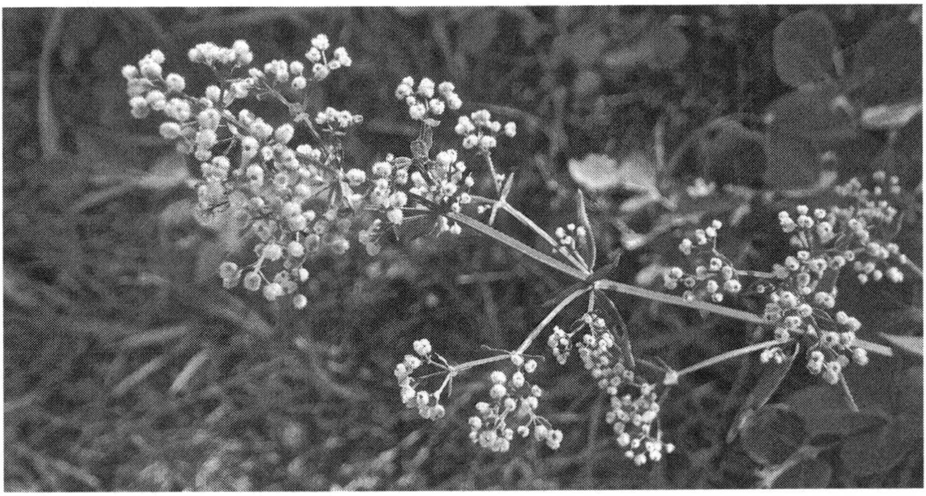

Northern Bedstraw

False Bedstraw or False Cleavers (*G. spurium*) contains saponins that show activity against both leukemia and breast cancer cell lines.

It is frequently used in Traditional Chinese Medicine, known as **ZHU YIN YIN**, **CHU YANG YANG**, or **ZHU YANG YANG**.

The plant has bitter, pungent and cold properties that enter the lungs, spleen, heart and kidney meridians.

Extracts have been shown to lower blood pressure without reducing heart rate.

Work by Orhan et al, *J Ethnopharm* 2012 141 220-7 identified anti-convulsant activity in mice studies, suggesting a rationale for traditional use in epilepsy.

A number of species contain asperuloside, which produces coumarin, and sweet hay scent. Asperuloside can be converted easily to prostaglandins, which are hormone-like compounds that stimulate the uterus and blood vessels, and is thus of interest not only to herbalists, but also the pharmaceutical industry.

Smooth Bedstraw has been investigated for anti-cancer and anti-malarial activity, and the ability to inhibit HIV reverse transcriptase, but with no activity. Grzybek et al, *Int J Pharmacog* 1997 35.

HOMEOPATHY

Galium aparine acts on the urinary organs, and is a diuretic for water retention, gravel and calculi. It has the power of suspending or modifying cancerous action. There is much clinical proof to confirm its use in cancerous ulcers and nodulated tumours of the tongue. It is a geriatric tonic.

Recent provings by Misha Roland at 30C potency give a few additional physical symptoms including itchiness, numbness, herpetic eruptions and sciatica. Mental symptoms include being overwhelmed, with changeable moods, and a pricking sensation accompanied by dreams of bees and wasps.

DOSE- 4-5 mls of tincture, three times daily. Mother tincture is made from the fresh plant in flower. For cancer of the tongue, which is tender and painful at night, use 20 drops every three hours. It can also be painted directly on the tumour.

PLANT OIL

Sweet scented bedstraw is sun infused, or prepared in a low temperature crockpot, with olive or canola oil in a ratio of 1:5. This could then be used for the vanilla like perfume notes or carrier oil for lymphatic massage blends.

The oil can be used to treat earache, gently warmed and a few drops applied. The fresh juice is also effective, and used in season or from frozen ice cubes.

Cleavers (*G. aparine*) has been analyzed and found to contain 22.3% hexadecanoic acid. An oil, prepared as above from freshly wilted aerial parts can be used for premenstrual sore breasts, or lumpy breasts associated with fibroadenoma. It is invaluable in cervical lymphatic nodes and swollen glands and in headaches associated with sinusitis.

ESSENTIAL OIL

Galium verum essential oil is composed of 29% cis-3-hexen-1-ol, 20% squalene, 10% diethylneglycol monomethyl ether, 7.8% benzyl alcohol, alpha terpineol and dozens of minor compounds.

HYDROSOL

The distilled water (of Cleavers), drank twice a day, helps the yellow jaundice. **CULPEPPER**

Lady Bedstraw water is distilled from the herb and root. It is warm and dry, comforting the head and brain and sight. It opens stoppages of the spleen and heals hernia, provokes urine, improves appetite, soothes the stomach, and with wormwood daily is good for ague, fits and fever.

BRUNSCHWIG

FLOWER ESSENCES

Cleavers is an excellent remedy for use by chiropractors. The kundalini energy up the spine is activated. It is also a good flower essence for those having trouble with their father image. Individuals who have difficulty studying or focusing on their chosen careers will likewise benefit from cleavers. **PEGASUS**

The elixir made from bedstraw flower helps in opening new internal passages of understanding and in focusing on the essential. A simple flower, it clarifies difficult moments and removes obstacles.

SCHNEIDER

Lady's Bedstraw (*G. verum*) essence is for new hope, ideas and grace. It provides freedom from the past. **ICELANDIC**

Lady's Bedstraw essence is for those suffering chronic worry, constant concerns and excruciating mental anguish. **MIRIANA**

PERSONALITY TRAITS

Think of cleavers, twisting upwards, and irritating as it does; the urethritis is often experienced from a genital infection lower down. The infection climbs further up the urethra, bladder to the kidneys and adrenal glands. Sexually transmitted diseases, as well as various viral infections will cause irritation, inflaming the prostate- even causing sterility!

The cleaver type is male, with an irritable bladder, and perhaps intermittent discharge and inflamed prostate.

Homeopathic miasma, relating to ancestral/cellular venereal infection, are treated well with cleavers.

Today, the conception of children to parents with a history of present day, or genetically passed on, venereal patterns leads to future generations of suffering.

Childhood eczema, or the sudden appearance of psoriasis can sometimes be traced to genetic pre-disposition.

On the positive side, the herbalist's job is the treatment of illness in early stages. Early detection of irritation, discharge or a local skin rash, calls for immediate treatment. The overuse of antibiotics often removes the symptoms, but fails to totally rid the body of the predisposition to later prostate or bladder cancer. Or more importantly, severe genetic skin disorders in future children can be avoided by early intervention. **DOROTHY HALL**

For me, it was easy to see cleavers' character emerge. I've always looked on cleavers as an herb that strives to please. It's a gentle, tender little soul that loves being loved and yearns to be needed.

One of the more obvious character traits is cleavers' determination to go home with you its tiny, velcro-like seeds latch onto shoes, socks, pants, shirt....you name it.

It's a bit on the insecure inside, I suppose, but it can't help it.

DEWEY

Cleavers has the quality of clinging as in holding on to. On a physical level it has to do with keeping together and holding in. On an emotional level, Cleavers has to do with maintenance, upholding and supporting. On a metaphysical level it can do the same thing. Cleavers would be useful if you wanted togetherness in a club or any group of people; it would help maintain their connectedness.

EVELYN MULDERS

Goose grass stands for ambiguity. Of a hazy, almost unimpressive appearance, goose grass proves itself to be a very strong and resistant plant.

It symbolizes ambiguity; of everything where appearance does not really tally with the true nature, with the essence of existence.

GRIMAUD

The negative aspects of cleavers arise from congested thoughts and irritability, especially over minor things. The person may be quite spiky, capricious, and fidgety. He may fret about the small things and may have an edgy, nervous, high-strung disposition. Urinary frequency often accompanies this nervous disposition. Cleavers helps to clear the moody, fearful, weepy, or self-pitying tendencies, bringing instead a contented, lighthearted approach to life.

CLARE GOODRICK-CLARKE

SPIRITUAL PROPERTIES

The finely edged stems remind us of the nerves. Cleavers has a considerable action on the nervous system. I have used it for head, spinal and nerve injuries.

The specific thing I learned was that Cleavers helps people who are irritated by little things, rather than—make similar to above after addition. That is what we would expect for a remedy that helps to filter out little materials.

Bedstraw is a Deer Medicine. These fine-boned, elegantly articulated, but somewhat nervous animals are associated with nerve medicine. The sharp edge of the stem seen in Cleavers is a signature pointing to the nerves, but it also reminds us of the fine, sharp-edged boney structure of the deer. **WOOD**

It is important to realize what it means when an inflorescence contains masses of small, regularly formed flowers... Many small regular flowers...are the expression of cosmic forces. **GROHMANN**

BOTANICA POETICA

Cleavers (*Galium aparine*)
Here's a very clingy weed
Sticks to clothes and other things
Its healing properties are great
Lymphatic drainage stimulate
It can tone and purify
Cleanse the blood, detoxify
Remove the burning of infection
Relieve you of an inflammation
Cools the heat, reduces fevers
Such is true of the plant, Cleavers
Known as Goosegrass, Bedstraw, Clives
Galium Aparine, besides
Use it as a birthing bed
Protects a pregnancy, it's been said
Drink the tincture for cystitis
Or a tea for hepatitis
If the neck glands start to swell
It's an herb that should work well
It's diuretic, it's lymphatic
Stimulates and clears the static
And if your skin is very dry
It's an herb you'll want to try
Make a poultice of this weed
It's got everything you need!
SYLVIA CHATROUX MD

ASTROLOGY

Venus rules the water economy of the body: the genitourinary system, the hormonal system, the gonads, the veins and the tongue. All kinds of kidney problems and dropsy come into her province. Cleavers removes the Saturn tendency to stagnation in the lymphatic system, cleansing and relieving the congestive and rigidifying tendencies of Saturn. It is beneficial to the bones, ruled by Saturn, as well as to the arteries, sinews, lymph and nerves. In fact, wherever there are long, tubular structures in the body—all ruled by Saturn—cleavers will clear them, flushing the toxins out through the urinary system.

Saturn governs eliminative functions, the bones, joints, ligaments, the spinal column, neck, limbs, and the skin. Cleavers streamlines the body, lessening edemas and restoring the clean lines of the facial contours where there was swelling, especially around the eyes. As a result of taking cleavers, the neck may be smooth, without the lumpy nodules of congested lymph nodes. **GOODRICK-CLARKE**

RECIPES

FRESH PLANT EXTRACTS- Take 1-2 teaspoons in water up to twice daily. This may be frozen in ice cube trays for out of season usage. Or combine fresh juice with 25% vodka as a preservative. This succus is taken 5-15 ml three times daily.

TINCTURE- 30-60 drops in water up to three times daily. For seizures, try 10-15 drops once or twice daily. For a fresh plant tincture, dry the plant for 24 hours in the shade, and then use a 30% alcohol mixture at 1:5; or use a 1:2 of really fresh herb at 50% for superior product.

FLUID EXTRACT- 4 mls three times daily.

DEODORANT- Take one handful of cleavers to one litre of water and bring to a boil. Simmer for 15 minutes. Leave to get cold, strain and bottle. Put in fridge, and apply to the armpits with a cotton batten. Repeat each week.

NOTE- Remember to use warm water with kidney complaints, and cold water with lymphatic or deep-seated problems.

CAUTION- Some herbalists recommend against using cleavers in hypotension, in cold conditions, or diabetes. The latter is due to an over stimulation of the adrenals, which in turn, can inhibit the effectiveness of insulin, and/or the diuretic effect.

It is not a hard and fast rule, just pay attention to individual needs of the client.

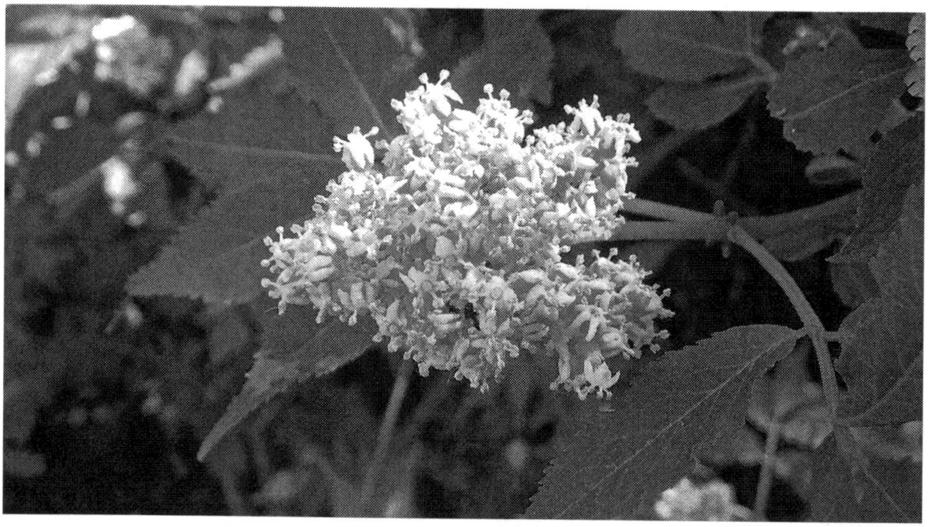

Red Elder flowers

RED ELDER
RED BERRIED ELDER
(*Sambucus pubens* Michx**)**
(*S. racemosa* ssp. *pubens* var. *arborescens*)
(*S. racemosa* ssp. *pubens* [Michx.] House**)**
BLACK ELDER
(*S. racemosa ssp. pubens*) var. *melanocarpa* [Gray] McMinn**)**
(*S. melanocarpa* A. Gray**)**
CANADIAN ELDER
AMERICAN ELDER
BLACK ELDER
(*S. canadensis* L.**)**
(*S. nigra ssp. canadensis* [L.] Bolli.**)**

BLUE ELDERBERRY
(S. nigra ssp. cerulea)
(*S. caerulea* Raf.)
(S. glauca)
EUROPEAN ELDER
BLACK ELDER
(*S. nigra* L.)
PARTS USED- leaves, flowers, stems, fruit

Around the boiling cauldrons
The old Elder trees stand.
The old Elders sing –
They sing of life, they sing of death,
They sing of the whole human race. **MANNHARDT 1877**

Hawthorn bloom and elder flowers
Will fill the house with evil powers. **M E S WRIGHT**

Sambucus is believed by some scholars to stem from the Greek **SAMBUKE**, an ancient lyre or harp made from elder wood, or from the Italian **SACKBUT** an early trombone. Both are highly unlikely.

It is probably from the Spanish **SACABUCHE** from **SACAR** meaning to draw, and **BUCHA**, a pipe, in reference to the use as a draw-tube for water.

The deeper meaning of the tree itself is Sambuca- the pipe of Pan- and it is his spirit blowing through this sacred tree that will heal and teach mankind.

In all ancient texts, elder is considered a panacea, "to be healed or cured by Pan, the deepest sacred power of forest".

Elder is derived from the Anglo-Saxon **AELD** or **ELLER** meaning fire kindler, referring to the hollow stems used as bellows for starting fires, or the Anglo-Saxon ***EALD*** meaning old, referring to longevity in those using elder in their diet. The Middle English verb **ELDEN** means, "to light a fire". The Romans called it **EBULUS** meaning, "to bubble out". Danewort (*S. ebulus*) is a poisonous species from the Mediterranean area.

More likely is that elder is derived from hulda, meaning hidden.

Or perhaps it is derived from Holla, the Great Goddess of Northern Europe. The tree was known in Old High German as **HOLUN TAR** meaning the tree of Holla. The fairy tale Frau Holle gathered by the Brothers Grimm, reveals her as the archetypal, well-meaning wise mother. Frau Holle was known as devil's grandmother by some, and the queen of the dwarves and elves by others.

Frau Holle is also a protector of souls and goddess of the dead.

Another possibility is the German folk names for the devil, **HOLDERLIN** and **HOLLABIRU**. This may have led to Holunder.

In Denmark, the Elder Mother, or **HYLLEMOER**, protected homes from illness and bad luck. Frisians buried their dead under the trees, and in Austria a cross of the wood was placed on the grave.

Elder is the letter R (ruis) in the Druid's tree alphabet, sacred to Hela, queen of the underworld. The Celts named it **CRANN TROIM**, the laden tree.

The tree is associated with Samhain and Venus.

European Elder is an introduced tree, while Sweet or Canadian Elder is usually found naturally no further west than Manitoba. Red Elder is native to Europe and western Asia, and cultivated since 1597. The crushed elder leaves were used to make green patterns on the freshly washed rock floors in Wales, to keep evil away.

Both *S. melanocarpa* and *S. pubens* are found in Alberta, the former with round, purple black berries, and the later with red, but sometimes white, or yellow fruit, in rocky places or higher elevations. All are hardy to zone 3.

Blue Elder is found on the other side of the continental divide, into Montana and further south. It plays a role in the creation myth of the Tsimschian.

In medieval times, the elder was associated with devils and witches. Spirits of the pagan dead, once called Helleder, were said imprisoned in elder wood. They would be transformed into avenging demons and haunt and persecute anyone who cut down an elder tree. If you fell asleep under an elder, you would have visions of Hel's underworld, which Christians converted into hell.

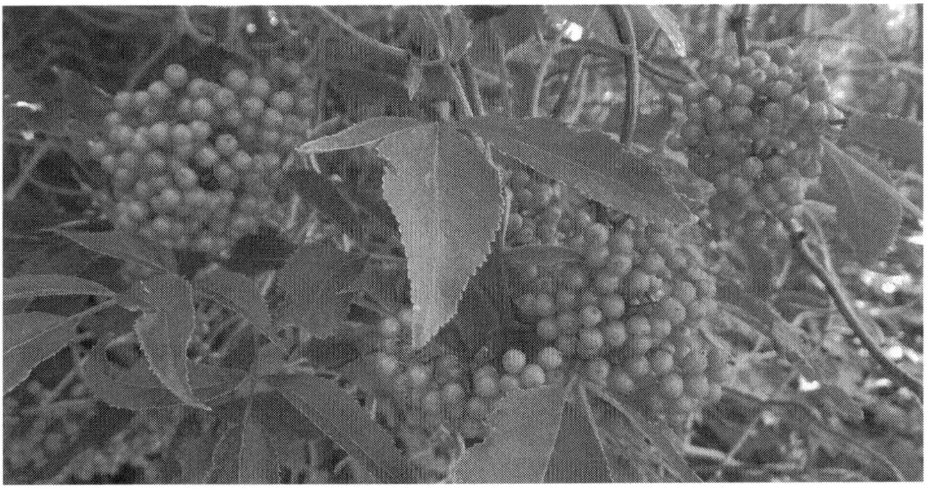

Red Elderberries

Early Christians also associated the sacred tree with the traitor Judas who hung himself after betraying Jesus.

Scandinavian folklore dedicated the tree to **HULDE**, the goddess of love, and **THOR**, the god of thunder. In the branches lived a dryad, **HYLDE-MOER**, the Elder Tree Mother. She would avenge any injury to the tree.

Elder is called Elle or Hyldemoer in Scandinavian and Danish lore. Huldafolk, meaning "hidden people" is the term for elder tree fairies in Iceland.

The Prussian Earth God and Latvian Prikaitis both lived under an Elder tree.

Elder is a member of the Honeysuckle family and a "first cousin" of snowberry.

Elderberry fruit was given to women by medieval herbalists and folk healers to help bring on menstruation.

Switches of the tree were used by herdsmen to insure their animal's safety. Elder twigs were spiked in rows of faba beans to prevent insect infestation.

In Irish folklore, falling asleep under the tree in flower may result in never awakening, as the fragrance can transport one to fairy realms.

Standing under the tree at Midsummer night, may give you a glimpse of the Fairy King and his entourage.

In the language of flowers, elderberry blossoms represent compassion, zeal, mercy, kindness and humility. Elder represents the birth date of May 20th. The number 5 is prominent, with five petals, five stamens and five sepals on the flowers; hanging on five stalks at the end of five stalklets.

Gypsies call it **YAKORI BENGESKRO**, meaning "devil's eye"; the black berries gathered on Midsummer Eve for protection against witchcraft.

Small pieces of the inner pith were cut, dipped in oil, and floated on a glass of water. It would direct its light towards any sorcerers lurking in the vicinity.

Natives of the prairies removed the semi-poisonous pith from the centre of stems to make flutes, whistles and straws. The dried roots were decocted for various respiratory infections, from flu to tuberculosis.

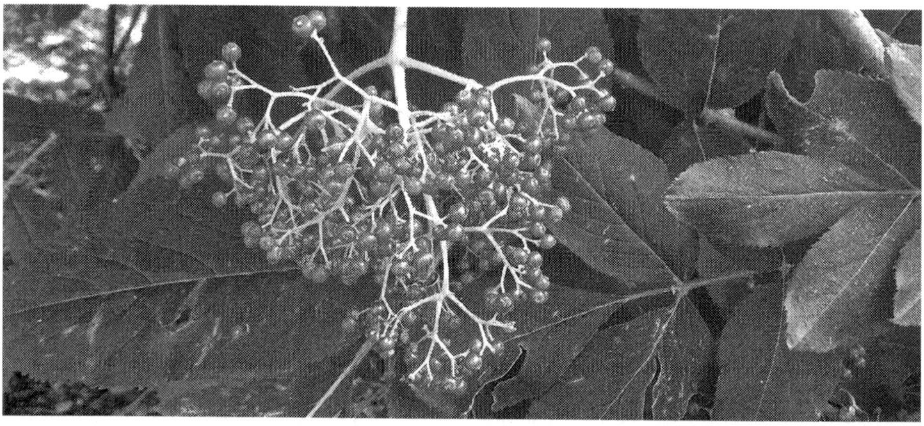

Sambucus racemosa

Many tribes used the bark of Red Elderberry (*S. racemosa*) to relieve toothache pain. The majority respected the bark's powerful emetic and purgative qualities, using only small amounts as needed. Simple infusions would cause vomiting and purging, and were used when patients were tired or with poor appetite.

In fact, *S. racemosa* bark is used in China, known as **SHAN SIU KIU**, as a purgative for cattle. Another name for the tree **SHU CHIN SHU** means, Muscle Relaxing Tree, or sometimes **HSU KU MU** meaning, Bone Connecting Wood. The flower is used for aching bones, knees, swollen feet and related cold pains.

The Thompson natives soaked their fresh salmon in berry juice before baking. The berries were mashed and dried into cakes, to be later reconstituted into fish head soups and other dishes. Caches of red elder berries have been found at archeological sites, dating hundreds of years old.

Unlike other elder, the root of this species is whitish.

Red Elderberry is known to the modern Gitksan of northern BC as **SGAN LOOTS'** meaning fruit plant.

They would not eat the fruits raw, but boiled them and made cakes dried for winter, combined with blue or black huckleberries. These dry berry cakes were kept in small boxes for winter, and used by the highest status members at feasts. The root bark was decocted and taken internally as an emetic for influenza.

The Saanich infused the bark to bring on birthing after delayed labour.

The Dena'ina of Alaska call it False Elder, Straight Plant, **CH'IHT'UN**, or that which pops inside, **BIK'DELTETL'A**, referring to the hollow stem which they arm with a piece of Birch Polypore (*Piptoporus betulinus*) as a type of pop gun toy for children.

The root of Red Elder was used as a medicine for cold, flu, high fever, and tuberculosis. The outer bark was peeled and thrown away. The remainder was boiled, squeezed and taken for infections or wash afflicted area. The leaves were boiled and used for tuberculosis.

The Haida call the berries **JITL'L** and the bush or wood, **STAAY** or **JITL'L**. They boiled the red berries for a long time and then mixed them with fish grease. The seeds were spit out.

The pith inside the stems was used to fasten flint arrow points onto shafts and as blunt tips for arrows, according to Nancy Turner.

The blue elderberry (*S. glauca*) bark was used by Haida, Saanich and Cowichan as a laxative.

Red Elder (*S. pubens*) berries, or **HUBU**, were picked in the fall by the Paiute, and spread out on a mat to dry. They were put in a woven sagebrush sack.

The berries were boiled, but not ground, into a type of soup.

The Blue Elderberry (*S. cerulea var. cerulea*) was eaten fresh or spread on rocks to dry by Paiute. The flowers and leaves were boiled as a vapor for steaming patients with colds or headaches. Flower tea was drunk for fever and to bring out measles.

In cases of blood poisoning, the affected limb was soaked in hot liquid from boiled leaves.

Hollowed branches were made into six hole flutes or holders for plugs of tobacco and tobacco-lime mixtures. Archeological sites in the eastern Mojave Desert contain arrow and dart shafts from elderberry canes.

Today, these elder stems can be used as spiles to tap birch trees. The pith is still utilized by watchmakers to help absorb grease and oil in workings. Biologists use it to grip minute biological specimens for microscope work. It is the softest, lightest, solid known with a specific gravity of 0.09. It is rubbed in science class to demostrate static electricity, in the form of pith balls.

The leaves have a very pungent odour that serve well as an insect repellent. Dry them and sprinkle on garden insects; they combine well with ox-eye daisy leaves. The leaves can be infused and used as a spray for aphids on houseplants or for garden aphids, rose mildew, greenfly and caterpillars. Combine elder leaves and yew needles as a spray for leaf miners.

Strong decoctions disperse ant nests overnight.

Water extracts of *S. racemosa* have been found an effective oviposition deterrent for the large cabbage butterfly.

The leaf rubbed on your skin and clothes lasts about a half hour to discourage mosquitoes.

Dairies traditionally hung the branches on the wall where cheese was made, to repel flies. A small branch hung on your clothes or in hair will save you from aggravating insects in the deep woods.

The flowers were eaten by first wrapping them in dough and frying in fat. Elderflower pancakes are traditional fare for the summer solstice in parts of Central Europe.

The un-opened flower buds are pickled like capers. In France, apples are packed in elder flowers to enhance the flavour and longevity of the fruit. Boiling the flowers in vinegar makes a black hair dye.

Elderflower extracts are found in various St. Ives Shampoo products.

The seedless berries make delicious jam. Both flowers and berries are used in wines. Country wines, produced by Cairn O'Mohr Winery use 8 tons of berries and 3 tons of flowers in their product. They have established plantations to expand their production. Another company, Balnakeil Wines, in Durness, produces five gallon batches of wine using elder, meadowsweet, mountain ash berry, nettle, dandelion, heather and birch leaf.

Elderflower water is famed for complexion and freckle removal. It combines well with yarrow and mint, for a refreshing footbath. Eau de Sareau, a commercial product, is made from one cup of the dried petals to one litre of hot water, and a little honey.

Black Elder (*S. nigra*) from Europe will grow on the prairies. Pearl Creek Farms, south of Melville, Saskatchewan is one good supplier of seedlings.

The purple elderberry (*S. canadensis*) contains anthocyanins that are more stable to light and heat than *S. nigra*, and could be further investigated for use in food colouring. Work by Inami et al, of Japan 1996 led to this finding.

Recent work by Ozgen et al, *Pharmacognosy Mag* 2010 6:23 looked at 14 successions of this shrub to optimize antioxidants, as well as phenolic and anthocyanin content of the purple-black berries for commercialization.

Both *S. canadensis* and *S. nigra* may die back in some prairie winters, but can be grown as shrubs.

Dr. O. Phelps Brown said of *S. canadensis*. "In warm infusions the flowers are diaphoretic and gently stimulant. In cold infusions they are diuretic, alterative, and cooling and may be used in all diseases requiring such action, as in hepatic derangements of children, erysipelas... the expressed juice of the berries, evaporated to the constituency of a syrup, is a valuable aperient and alterative; one ounce of it will purge... the flowers and expressed juice of the berries have been beneficially employed in scrofula, cutaneous diseases, syphilis, rheumatism, etc."

Several native tribes, including the Algonquin used *S. canadensis*, along with black and white spruce and Wintergreen (*Gaultheria procumbens*), as a blood purifier, after boiling them together for several hours.

The bark was taken by Meskwaki women to help uterine contractions and quicken labor. The Seneca used green shoot bark steep in water to treat measles.

Onondaga aboriginal peoples scraped bark and made a warm poultice that was applied to the forehead for migraine headaches.

The Seneca also used the green young shoots for heart disease, collecting them before July. The pith sponge was removed and steeped for three hours, no longer.

Both Seneca and Cayuga used steeped blossom tea to sponge newborns as part of a new birth ritual. Mother's milk was reserved for eyes, ears and nose.

The flower tea of red elderberry helps to calm asthmatic symptoms, as well as stomach and liver irritation. The fruit juice is somewhat laxative, and soothing in cases of nephritis.

All ripe berries are safe and edible when cooked, and the seeds discarded. The raw berry may cause nausea in some people.

Elderflowers are toxic to turkeys. A flower tea discourages mold, and makes a handy, organic spray for greenhouse or garden varieties. Elder leaf infusions, made by soaking overnight, protects rose and other flowers from blight, as well as deter aphids and caterpillars from fruit bushes.

MEDICINAL

CONSTITUENTS- *S. racemosa* berries- contain cyanidin-3-sambubioside 5-glucoside (like *S. nigra*), as well as cyandin-3-p-coumaryl sambubioside 5- glucoside and two acylated glucosides of cyanidin.
The flowers are comprised of elderin, various oils, triterpenes, malates of potash and lime.
Root and bark- choline, ursolic acid
S. canadensis fruit- various anthocyanins including cyanidin 3-[6-{p-coumaryl)-2-(xylosyl)-glucoside]-5-glucoside and sambucin, various amino acids, minerals, 2.4% fat. Sambunigrin in unripe berries and other parts of plant.
seed- 32% fat, resin, tannins
bark- baldrianic acid
shoot- morroniside
S. nigra fruit- various anthocyans, including cyanidine-3-glycoside (40%), cyanidine-3-sambubioside (44-46%), cyanidine-3-sambubioside-5-glucoside (10%), and cyanidine-3,5-diglucoside (3%). The berries are rich in Vit A, flavonoids, fruit sugars, calcium, thiamin and niacin.
Seeds- cyanogenic glycosides including holocalin, prunasin, sambunigrin and zierin.
flowers- flavonoids (3%) including rutin, isoquercitin, astragalin, quercitin and kaempferol; phenolic acids including chlorogenic acid, p-coumaric acid, and caffeic acid, essential oil, triterpenes such as alpha and beta amyrin, ursolic acid, mucilage, minerals especially potassium, and sterols.
bark and leaves- rutin, beta sitosterol, lupeol, tannins, cyanogenic glycosides like sambunigrin; baldrianic acid, sambucine, valerianic acid, potassium nitrate and variable amounts of hydrocyanic acid. The bark contains phytohemagglutins and lectins.

Elderflower is the ideal herb for breaking colds and flu. It combines well with peppermint and yarrow in a hot infusion to induce sweating and break the fever. In TCM this is known as dispersing of wind heat.

The removal of toxins through the skin is especially useful in eruptive childhood diseases such as mumps, chickenpox, and measles, to bring out the rash and speed recovery.

In TCM, this would mean clearing heat, relieving toxicity, drying dampness and venting rashes.

Cooling and drying, it is indicated in weeping eczema where skin separates and discharge forms pus and crusts, as well as indolent ulcers with boggy borders that will not heal in. In this case drink cool.

To treat catarrhal inflammation such as sinusitis and hay fever, combine with yarrow. It is most useful when phlegm is white or turning yellow.

For catarrhal deafness, combine with plantain, and with linden flowers for persistent or nervous coughs.

Elderflower's anti-inflammatory action has been demonstrated in work by Mascolo et al, *Phytotherapy Research* 1987 1.

Elderflower contains a natural antispasmodic that relieves bronchial spasms, as well as menstrual cramps; and increases milk flow in new mothers.

Elderflower infusions, at body temperature, treat various kidney and bladder ailments, including acute nephritis, renal liathisis, and cystitis with water retention. The removal of heat and clearing of toxins aids arthritis, rheumatism and gout.

Liver heat with symptoms of sore throat, red eyes, lung abscess and sores on upper body and face are relieved.

Hot infusions are best for diaphoretic and stimulating qualities, as well as expectorating properties. Cold infusions are diuretic.

Elder flowers are cooling, immune building, slightly blood-thinning, soothing, mildly stimulating and slightly tonic, according to Matthew Wood.

The fresh flowers are a stimulating diaphoretic and used for pale, bluish persons with weak peripheral circulation. The dry flowers are a sedative diaphoretic that reduce heat, open the pores, and disperse blood in people with dry, irritable red skin of the cheeks of the face and "cheeky" parts of the body.

Matthew lists a constitutional type for the flowers. It is the great infant remedy; for infants with blue, pale swelling across the nose, red, dry, irritated skin of the cheeks; "opens the tubes and pores," lubricates the skin, improved respiration, digestion and kidney function.

Also use for conditions where there are both stagnant fluids and blood, hence pale, blue swelling or where the skin is dry, harsh and red.

Methanol extracts of the flowers inhibit biosynthesis of various cytokines *in vitro*, including interleukin-l alpha, interleukin-l beta, and TNF-alpha. Yesilada et al, *J Ethnopharm* 1997 58:1.

Elderflowers are soothing and relaxing to the nerves, helping anxiety and depression. Hot infusions at night are good at the onset of infections in children.

I often mix elderflower syrup, in sparkling water for a refreshing, cooling summer drink. Rekorderlig, an elderflower flavoured pear cider, is a summertime favorite of my wife Laurie.

It is good for swollen tonsils and lymphatic swelling, taken in cold water.

Chlorogenic acid is found in elderflowers and numerous other herbs. It has been suggested via *in vitro* studies to help prevent atherosclerosis and free radical damage, as well as act as anti-tumour agent.

Elderflower combines well with Echinacea, and cleavers for damp heat rash, with mullein leaf and red clover blossom for wind heat coughs, and with chrysanthemum flowers for strong heat effusion with sore throats, and cough.

Elderflowers contain water-soluble constituents that directly stimulate muscular glucose metabolism and promote insulin secretion from pancreatic cells. Gray et al, *Journal of Nutrition* 2000 130:1.

Work at Tufts University identified 4 anthocyanins in the berry that protect endothelial cells that line arteries, from oxidative stress.

Streptococcus infection of the skin and throat is relieved by berry juice. Other skin conditions, including eczema, boils, skin itching and sensitive skin all respond to topical application as fomentation or salves.

Ointments from elder leaves have shown good results in bruises, sprains and skin tumours.

The leaves when fresh can be applied to boils to disperse heat.

Extracts from the Black Elderberry (*S. nigra*) have shown in clinical studies to possess very effective anti-viral activity. Sambucol, one common extract from Israel, has shown activity against influenza A and B.

The product combines Black elderberry and red raspberry extracts, with echinacea and bee propolis. Barak et al, *Eur Cytokine Netw* 2001 12.

A double-blind, placebo-controlled trial of 60 patients with flu-like symptoms found those taking elderberry syrup had reduction of symptoms four days sooner than placebo group. Zakay-Rones et al, *J Int Med Res* 2004 32:2.

Work by Dr. Madeleine Mumcuoglu found elderberry disarms the neuraminidase enzyme flu viruses use to penetrate healthy cells. This mechanism of action is used by both H5N1 Bird Flu and West Nile Flu; suggesting black elderberry extract use for immune protection in viral epidemics.

Bill Roschek et al, *Phytochem* 2009 August 12 found elderberry extracts effective against the HINI virus. The IC50 of one compound was 0.36 uM compared to Tamiflu at 0.32 uM. The extract appears to bind and prevent the virus from entering cells, at least *in vitro*.

It appears to modulate Th1 response, associated with inflammation. Work by Waknine-Grinberg et al, *Planta Med* 2009 75:6 found the animal response to leishmania positive, and yet it aggravated and intensified induced malaria.

A placebo-controlled, double-blind study of elderberry extract was conducted in Panama by Zakay-Rones et al and reported in the *Journal of Alternative and Complementary Medicine* in 1995. It showed that those volunteers treated had fewer symptoms, recovered quicker and produced more anti-viral antibodies than controls, to an outbreak of influenza B. The seeds possess potent anti-viral activity and should be included in the final product.

Elderberry appears to have some potential in HIV-1 infection. It binds to viral glycoproteins other than gp41, the binding site for enfuvirtide. Fink et al, *Antivir Chem Chemother* 2009 19:6.

Eva Aschenbrunner mentions the use of elderberry for shingles, a painful herpes zoster viral episode.

Work by Sauter and Wolfensberger found *S. racemosa* berries cytotoxic, with no replication of the avian influenza virus after a three-day screening.

The berries of *S. nigra, S. canadensis*, and *S. glauca* contain a sugar complex called 3-rhamnoglucoside. This helps the eye adjust to light levels and changes, and is considered useful in preventing optical ageing.

Berry juice from all three is used as part of body detoxification programs. Care is noted due to extreme alkalizing effect.

Elderberry is effective in the treatment of chronic venous insufficiency and lymphoedema. Whether due to infection or surgery (radical mastectomy), lymph fluid accumulates, extremities swell, causing pain. Wadworth and Faulds, *Drugs* 1992 reviewed the efficacy of a semi-synthetic flavonoid, hydroxy-ethylrutoside, in venous insufficiency and related disorders.

Black elderberry shows hypoglycemic, hypolipidemic and anti-oxidant activity in diabetic-induced rats. Ciocoin et al, *Rev Med Chir Soc Med Nat Isai* 2008 12:3.

The flowers increase glucose uptake and reduce fat accumulation in lab *in vivo* studies, suggesting modulation of glucose and lipid metabolism. Bhattacharya S et al, *J Agric Food Chem* 2013 61(146):11033-40.

An agglutinin exhibits activity against human colon cancer cells in work by Dali'Olio et al, 2000 and 2001; and Fernandez-Rodriguez et al, 2000.

Black Elder bark is still the treatment of choice in France for some cases of grand mal and petit mal epilepsy.

It is used for pyleonephritis, urethritis, cystitis and urinary retentions; as well as cleansing the bladder of urinary gravel.

Young bark from Elder is used in tincture form for asthmatic conditions and croup in children.

Anti-viral activity from branch tip extract of *S. racemosa* was found by McCutcheon et al, *J Ethnopharm* 1995 49 101-110. The berries show anti-fungal and anti-bacterial activity. The bark of *S. racemosa* ssp. *pubens* shows activity against MRSA, or methicillin resistant *Staphylococcus aureus*. *J Ethnopharm* 1992 37 213-223.

An extract of elderberry leaves, St. John's wort and soapwort has been found to inhibit the influenza and herpes simplex virus in the lab.

Bergeron et al, found methanol extracts of *S. canadensis* leaves effective against *Candida albicans*. Dicloromethane extracts of the root leaves, flowers and shoots showed biological effect against fungi, *Bacillus subtilis* and *E. coli*. Water extracts showed no activity.

Both ether and saline extracts of the leaves showed activity against both gram positive and negative bacteria. Michael Moore suggests dry elder leaves are a very effective diaphoretic. Stephen Buhner, in *Herbal Antivirals*, notes the anti-viral, anti-bacterial and anti-inflammatory compounds are stronger in the leaf, stem and roots. Fresh leaf tinctures relax the nervous system and cause diaphoresis. "The leaves, like peach leaves, are a very reliable nervine. That is, they relax the nervous system. That is why the herb was used for epileptic fits, and various dementias and uncontrollable movements, by both European and American herbalists for centuries. Dosage of the fresh leaf tincture runs from 5 to 10 drops, taken no more than each hour."

Thole et al, *J Med Food* 9:4 found extracts of this species inhibit a marker in the promotion stage of carcinogenesis.

A new neolignan glycoside has been recently isolated from the root bark of *S. racemosa.* It is interesting, in that its structural relationship is similar to the liver protecting compounds found in Milk Thistle.

In Traditional Chinese Medicine, the leaves, stem and roots are used in decoction for traumatic injuries, fractures, arthralgia, and for promoting callus formation and muscle and sinew healing. External bathing, is combined with decoctions taken internally.

Water extracts from the leaves of *S. pubens* show anti-mycobacterium activity.

Elderberry bark provides sialic acid specific lectins that are used to study this acid on the surface of cancer cells. Fischer et al, *Glycoconjugate J* 1995 12.

A lectin related protein, SNLRP, from the bark, is a novel ribosome inactivating protein with an inactive B chain, devoid of carbohydrate binding activity.

The bark may be emetic when taken as a decoction. Taken in small doses it acts on the lymph, colon, kidneys, causing loose stool and urination. The bark of our Elderberry contains sambucine, a nauseating alkaloid.

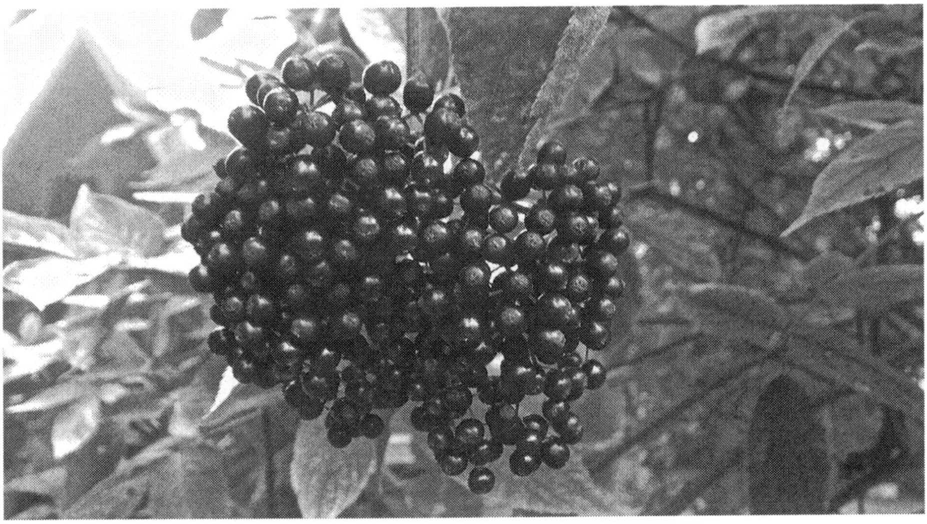

Black Elder *(S melanocarpa)*

The dried inner bark may be combined with flowers for edema, nephritis, urinary tract infections with sand in urine that passes.

The stems of *S. sieboldiana*, from China, Japan, and Korea, contain several compounds that appear to inhibit bone resorption via activity stimulated by parathyroid hormone activity.

Vanillic acid, vanillin, and coniferyl alcohol all showed significant inhibitory effect on bone resorption. Huiying Li et al, *Bio Pharm Bulletin* 1998 21:6.

HOMEOPATHY

Sambucus canadensis is of great value in decreasing water retention.

A proving of fresh flowerbuds, flowers, young twigs and leaf tincture (20-50 drops) was undertaken by Dr. Ubelacker. The following symptoms appeared: Drawing in the head, with anxious dread; flushed and blotched face; dryness and sensation of swelling of the mucous membranes of the mouth, pharnyx, larnyx, and trachea; frequent and profuse flow of clear urine; heaviness and constriction of the chest; palpitation of the heart, pulse rose to 100, and remained until perspiration ensued; sharp darting rheumatic pains in the hands and feet; exhaustion and profuse perspiration, which relieved all symptoms.

DOSE- Fluid extract- up to one teaspoon three times daily. Not sure, but mother tincture of *S. nigra* is prepared from either equal parts of the flowers and leaves; or the inner bark, depending upon whom you read. The 3X potency is used in Sambucus Compound manufactured by Weleda. Proving was by self experimentation of Uebelacker with tincture in 1880s.

Sambucus nigra is used for glottal spasms, profuse night sweats, pulmonary tuberculosis, asthma and various catarrhs. Knot in stomach, bowels feel bruised. Thigh tendons too short.

Cramps and pains, sweating all over. Worse from fruit and coffee.

It is also used for irrational fears, arising particularly at night. Fright and fear of suffocation, delusions of having to share bed with someone, of being forsaken by doctor. Dreams of flying, cats, meeting old friends, or people not seen for years.

DOSE above. First proving by Hahnemann, then self experiment by Lembke with tincture. Proving by Teresa Bernard with five females at 30c in 1998, and poisoning effects from leaves and flowers observed by Christison in 1830s.

[Black Elderberry] has a particular affinity for the lungs and kidneys. It is a powerful cleanser, acting on the respiratory and urinary systems and the skin. A keynote indication is when an individual sleeps into an attack, waking suddenly with mental anxiety, asthma, dyspnea or perspiration.

The person may have dreamed of suffocation and then awakened to find themselves in a suffocative attack.

GOODRICK-CLARKE

GEMMOTHERAPY

Black Elder bud macerate is used for muscle and acute joint pain, as well as rheumatism. It helps elimination of toxins in obesity and relieves hemorrhoids.

DOSE- 20-30 drops three times daily of 1DH glycerine macerate.

ESSENTIAL OILS

CONSTITUENTS- *S. nigra* flowers- trans-3,7-dimethyl1-1; 3,7-octatrien-3-ol (13%); palmitic (11.3%), linalool (3.7%),cis-hexanl, cis- and trans-rose oxides, nerol oxides, hotroenol, nonanal; as well as small amounts of caprin, caproin, and caprylin.

From the dried flowers, an essential oil is steam distilled. It is solid at room temperature, with the consistency of butter. It has a peculiar, intensely honey-like, and unpleasantly animal odour. Melting point is 47 degrees Celsius.

An absolute is made, by solvent extraction. Both are used extensively in various cosmetic products for their superb moisturizing effect.

The scent of *S. canadensis* flowers is more pleasant, resembling muscatel. The related *S. racemosa* has sweet smelling flowers, free of any fishy undertones common to other related species.

SEED OIL

Oil has been extracted from the seeds of *S. racemosa*, and yields 22-28%.

It has a very large proportion of palmitic acid (23%), 45% oleic acid, and 25% linoleic acid. It contains 30% hexabromides and has an iodine value of 177; saponification value of 180 with 1.48% unsaponified.

The pulp of the fruit contains about 4% oil, with an iodine value of 81.4-98.6.

The Canadian elder (*S. canadensis*) seed oil yields 22-28%; with an iodine value of 175, and specific gravity of 0.9351.

The seed oil is composed of 53% linoleic acid, 4% oleic, and 5.8% palmitic acid.

HYDROSOL

Take ten pounds of elderflowers, free from stalk to every five gallons of water and distill.

Little oil is realized, but the water is valuable in a variety of cosmetics for skin conditions, as well as clearing freckles, and effects of sunburn.

Viaud considers the distilled hydrolat very important for treating asthma and associated bronchial and pulmonary conditions.

Catty suggests the distilled water may be helpful as a compress in arthritis and sports injuries, as well as a circulatory stimulant, mild diuretic and kidney specific.

She recommends the water for beverage punch and ice cubes as well as desserts and other sweets.

Brunschwig suggested elder bud and leaf water for dropsy and broken bones. The flower water was reserved for trembling of hands, tertiary fevers, head pain, pimples, to comfort the stomach and remove cataracts from the eye. *Book of Distillation* 1530.

FLOWER ESSENCES

Elderflower essence is a mental rejuvenator. It is excellent after setbacks and combines well with fireweed; restoring confidence in the future; and helping to set positive goals.

It mellows the aggressive, and gives courage to the meek. It helps the weighing of options, and those who tend to procrastinate. It is also helpful for those who have difficulty with authority figures.

MOUNT JULIUS

Elder flower essence (*S. racemosa*) helps contract overly expanded states of being; helps one view life from the centre, rather than from the periphery. **ALASKA (RESEARCH)**

Red Elder flower essence helps us to remember that we already are Light. Everything else is like shadows cast by passing clouds.

TREE FROG

Red Elder essence helps increase joy and child-like anticipation of forthcoming events. **MIRIANA**

Elder (*S. canadensis*) flower essence is infused in the radiance of a summer full moon. It holds the joy and exuberance, the magic and mystery of the plant spirits. It offers protection on the etheric and spiritual planes. Essence of starlight! **WOODLAND**

Essence of Elder is used to promote feelings of self worth. It is especially useful in times of transformation and change and is good for fretful children. **GIFFORD**

SPIRITUAL PROPERTIES

Many folk traditions suggest that the elder was used for Christ's crucifixion; and perhaps, as well, the tree that Judas used to hang himself. The fungus on the tree is often called Judas' Ear.

Gypsy custom forbade the use of wood on campfires. The Russians believed the tree drove away evil spirits. Bohemians went to the tree with a spell to take away fever. Sicilians thought that sticks of the wood killed serpents and drove away robbers. Serbs introduced Elder into the wedding ceremonies for good luck. The English believed that the Elder was never struck with lightning. A twig was tied in three or four knots and carried to ward off rheumatism.

It was also believed that the Elder bush, trimmed into the form of a cross, and planted on a new grave would keep the soul beneath happy- if it blossomed. The green branches were also buried in graves to protect the dead from witches and other evils.

All of the above uses make us ponder the levels of awareness.
Ed Smith, of the Herb Pharmacy says "elder is a virtual condominium of plant devas". **PRAIRIE DEVA**

Elderberry's keyword is patience. It allows for the capacity to wait and know that all things are in God's time. Elderberry is the herb of collective consciousness. **EVELYN MULDERS**

The lesson of the elder is a difficult one. Not only are you asked to accept the inevitability of your own death, but you are also asked the far more personal and potentially embarrassing question- how might you be fated to be remembered, both for good and ill, were you to die today? In the dark days of winter, elder presents us with a mirror in which we must see ourselves truly reflected if we are to die with dignity and without regrets. **GIFFORD**

Individuals who are easily frightened or those who have a history of fright will benefit from this plant. The person in need of the remedy may visibly tremble. Sometimes the fright has a close connection to losing a parent (usually a mother) at a very early age. In *Cymbeline*, Shakespeare mentions the tree as a symbol of grief. Both asthma—holding on to the breath—and edema—holding on to water in the body—represent the psychological need to hold on to something very dear, and both are a somatization of the deep fear occasioned by sudden loss. As a result of trauma, there may be delusions and dreams with visions of horrible faces.

The elder essence helps individuals to mature into their own independence and realize that a parent cannot always be available to take care of them. It allows them to shape their own lives, making decisions for themselves, and to accept that in the great mysteries of life and death, we cannot always know why someone lives and another does not.

Lives can become stuck if there is too much fear. The essence works on the fourth chakra, the heart, and reminds us that love drives out fear. The essence also works on the fifth chakra, the throat and lungs. Fear stifles the breath. Articulating fears may help individuals to come to understanding. **GOODRICK-CLARKE**

PERSONALITY TRAITS

The [Elderflower] patient has acute influenza with fever and nasal obstruction and a history of recurring rhinitis and sinusitis. **ROSS**

As far as elderberry is concerned, there are three sorts of people: those gripped by nausea as soon as they smell elder, even from a distance; those who don't mind elder soup; and those who are not only capable of eating raw elderberries with milk and sugar but actually look forward to doing so. **JURGEN DAHL**

Sambucus canadensis fears impending danger and accidents. Constantly anxious, they are always on edge, startled easily, nervously perspiring from every trifle. Small things become large and frightful, including every small symptom. **VERMEULEN**

Elder's nature is discerning, discriminating and protective. **CRUDEN**

There are times when I want to be stained, marked all over by berry wine, baptized, mouth, fingers, chin and neck, between my toes, up my legs like the wine-makers of Jerez who walk round and round in tubs of berries all day, who return then to their homes at night wreathed in berry halos, heady with ripe flower bouquets dizzy with bees, their bodies painted, perfumed by purple sun syrup, their breath elderberry delicious. **PATTIANN ROGERS**

Probably one of the most important biochemicals is in the mature black fruit of the elderberry. It is a rhamnose sugar complex. It increases the efficiency of the metabolism in the avian eye, aiding visual acuity in the transition zones from darkness to light and vice-versa. This sugar is much sought after by songbirds in their north-south migrations of the global garden. **BERESFORD-KROEGER**

MYTHS AND LEGENDS

Stone and Elder disputed which should give birth to man. Stone said that if she gave birth to humans, they would live a long time, but if Elder gave people birth, they would die soon.

A great giant was lurking nearby and listening. He came nearer and touched Elder and told her that she would first give birth to man. So Elder gave birth to a child.

This is the reason why people do not live very long and why elders grow on graves. **GUILLET**

In the beginning there was only one elder tree, that grew far away to the east towards the rising sun in a den of rattlesnakes, and as the wind swayed its branches they sang together day and night to the two women of the star people that watched over it. Now there was one Wek-Wek, the Falcon, grandson of Coyote man who made the world, who had heard its music and wanted to possess the tree. So he journeyed to its home, and after many importunities persuaded these two heavenly ladies to part with some of its root, that from it many cuttings could be made and all the world could hear its melodies. The old Indians say that in some parts of the country there are still such trees to be found that give off sweet music at night- if one should listen very carefully, for so it used to be. **MERRIAM**

The Tsimschian said that in the beginning of the world, the elderberry argued with a boulder over who would give birth to the human race. Raven instructed the elderberry to give birth first, so it was the elderberry from which human beings arose. The Tsimschian apparently felt it necessary to explain why people did not live very long, and they understood that elderberries did not live long either. In contrast, boulders did. If the boulder had won the battle, people would live a long time; but as it was, the elderberry won, so the people die .

TAMRA ANDREWS

ASTROLOGY

All respiratory diseases come under the dominion of Mercury, the messenger, which governs the relationship between the inner and the outer being.

The lungs are a frontier between life forces in the outer world and the inner body, where the breath, oxygen, prana, chi is processed… Anxiety and fear can interrupt this process…those in this state must learn the art of letting go, a process of coming to trust the universe and their own responses to it. The skin is another organ in which the inner and outer world meet. Asthma and skin ailments can often alternate; if eczema is suppressed with steroids, the person will develop asthma, forming another vicious cycle. **GOODRICK-CLARKE**

BOTANICA POETICA

Elder
(*Sambucus nigra/S. canadensis*)
Here we have Black Elder Tree
Berry, Bark, Flower, Leaf
Each with special property
It's got a long time history
The Elder Tree is quite renown
Thousands of years it's been around
Folklore says where it is found
Is the doorway to the Underground!
The flower is for a cold or flu
Opens up the bronchial tube
Fights catarrh and helps with croup

A healthy sweat you could induce
Use the leaf for muscle pain
Apply a poultice to your strain
Rheumatic ailments you could tame
Elder leaves for chilblains
Beware Sambucus if it's Red!
There's a tip you shan't forget
Tell your sister and a friend
Red Elder you would quick regret
With the berries make a juice
There's Vitamin C in there too
Purify the blood for you
Boost immunity and fight the Flu!
SYLVIA CHATROUX

RECIPES

OUTER BARK DECOCTION- Scrape off the outer bark of 1-2 year old branches. Cut small and dry. Steep 2 ounces in 5 ounces boiling water for 48 hours. Give small mouthful when epileptic seizures threaten.

FLOWER INFUSION- Steep flowers in hot water for ten minutes. Cool. Soak in cotton ball and apply to styes and blepharitis.

TINCTURE- FLOWER- 15-30 drops as needed, made from dry flowers at 1:5 and 40% alcohol, or preferably from fresh flowers at 1:3 and 60%. Fresh leaf tincture uses same ratio.

CAUTION- Use elderflowers with caution for weak, cold, qi vacuous patients.

STANDARDIZED BERRY EXTRACT- up to 4000 mg daily in three divided doses containing 28% anthocyanins.

BERRY SYRUP- 1-2 tbsp twice daily. Use two cups fresh berries or one cup dried to 2 litres of water and 20 cups of sugar. Soak dried berries in water overnight in fridge. Bring to boil and reduce by half. Remove from heat, strain, throw away berry remains and return liquid to medium heat and stir in sugar. If you use 10 cups of sugar (still a lot) add 20% alcohol to preserve after cooling.

ANTIVIRAL ELDER RECIPE- powder one cup dried elder leaves and ½ cup of dried stems. Place in 2.5 litres of water and bring to boil. Reduce to simmer and cook until reduced by two-thirds. Remove and let cool. Press decoction through cloth, add one ounce elderberry syrup above, and one ounce each of fresh elder leaf tincture and fresh stem bark tincture. Return to heat and add enough sugar to bring up to 65% and let cool. **BUHNER**

OIL OF SWALLOWS- (also called *oleum viride*, green oil, or oil of elder)

Take one part of bruised, fresh elder leaves in three parts of cold pressed flaxseed or canola oil. Let stand for two weeks shaking daily. Strain. Use for bruises, sprains, chilblains, and wounds. Use low temperature crock pot if weather is inclement.

ELDERFLOWER OINTMENT- Take equal parts by weight of fresh flowers and canola oil. The flowers are heated until crisp, in the oil. This is cooled and sufficient beeswax is added to make smooth. Use on chapped hands, or hands and feet affected by cold.

POLLEN- When drying flowers on screen, catch the pollen that falls below and use in cosmetics.

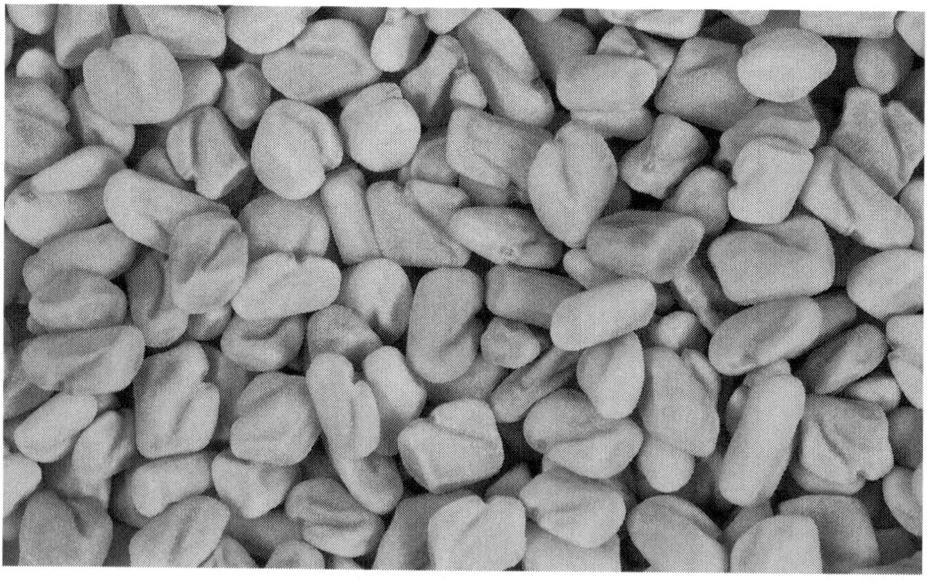

Fenugreek seeds

FENUGREEK
(*Trigonella foenum-graecum* L.)
PARTS USED- leaves, seeds

Widow Brown she had no children,
Though she loved them very dear;
So she took some Vegetable Compound,
Now she has them twice a year. **LYDIA PINKHAM**

May you tread in peace on the soil where it gave new strength, and fearless mood, and gladiators, fierce and rude,
Helbah (Fenugreek) grows! **MIDDLE EAST GREETING**

Foenum graecum is Latin for Greek Hay, a reference to the use of the plant in Greece to scent inferior hay. Trigonella is from the Greek **TREIS** for three, and **GONU** meaning angle or corner, and referring to the triangular appearance of the flowers.

Fenugreek is an annual, knee-high legume with considerable promise for the future on the prairies. It is a nitrogen-fixing crop, with high protein fodder. The yellow white sweet pea-like flowers are tinged with violet at the base.

The 10-20 seeds in each beaked pod are smooth, very hard and irregular in shape. Yields of 550-900 pounds per acre can be expected on the prairies.

One hundred and ten frost-free days are needed for full seed maturity, but the long, hot summer days of northern Alberta shorten this considerably. Fortunately it will germinate in cold soil, and needs about 35 pounds of seed sown per acre.

Fenugreek is an ancient crop, having been found at archeological sites in Iraq dated 4000 BC.

It is of Oriental origin, but has long been cultivated in the Mediterranean region, and more recently in North America.

The Egyptians used it as a component of **KUPHI**, incense of fumigation and embalming; with seeds found in the tomb of King Tut. The seeds were soaked in water until they swelled into a thick paste. The perfume **TELINON** was based on fenugreek seed, from the Greek **TELIS**.

In 71 AD, the Romans lay siege to Jerusalem. The trapped Jews boiled vast amounts of fenugreek, which because of its high pectin content, turns into a potent jelly when it cools.

The defenders poured the boiled fenugreek on the walls and rocks surrounding the city, making them too slippery for the Romans to climb.

The Egyptian Ebers papyrus (1500 BC), records the use of fenugreek for burns; "When the body is rubbed with it, the skin is left beautiful without any blemishes". The seeds were used in ancient Egypt to induce childbirth. The leaf is one of the chief ingredients in Kuphi, the renowned oil of anointment.

The Greeks used the plant to improve the roundness of women's breasts, and to stimulate the flow of breast milk. This makes sense in light of the fact that fenugreek, as well as alfalfa and asparagus, contains L-arginine that promotes release of human growth hormone from the pituitary.

Work by Turkyilmaz et al, *J Alt Comp Med* 2011 17:2 found increased breast milk with lower birth rate loss in first week and regaining original birth weight faster than placebo.

Work by Shim et al, *Chem Biodivers* 2008 51:9 found methanol extracts of isolated dioscin and saponin I stimulate pituitary secretions in rats.

The Greek name Keratitis is derived from the word Keras meaning horn, in reference to the shape of the seed.

Women in Libya and Eritrea eat fenugreek seeds to gain weight; while the Yemenites have, for centuries, used the seeds, to reduce blood sugar in a puree of boiled seeds with onion and meat called **HELBA**.

In the Middle East, they are boiled, and served as a vegetarian high protein main dish. Mohammed was a fan. "If you knew the value of fenugreek, you would pay its weight in gold".

Charlemagne ordered it grown in France in the 9th century, and Benedictine monks spread it throughout Europe.

Girls, from the Czech Republic, wear tiny bunches of fenugreek around their necks to attract young men's attention.

The seeds can be easily sprouted, and make for a tasty addition to salads, sandwiches and soups. They provide a rich source of natural vitamins, lecithin and iron, including the difficult to obtain B_{12}.

Fenugreek seed is used as a seasoning in coffee and vanilla extracts, chutney, tobacco flavouring, artificial maple syrup and of course, roasted for curry. Flavour fractions are used for flor-sherry wine in France, give unique aroma to sake, as well as enhance soy sauce, sugar molasses, and barley malt.

They are added to halva, a sweet Mid Eastern sweetmeat treat and condiment called hilbeh. In Yemen, it is mixed with other spices in zhug that is put on top of stews. Armenians add it to chili and garlic for chemen, used to spice beef dishes. Dry roasting adds depth of flavor.

In Arabian Medicine, it is used "for alluring roundness of the female breast".

Roasted seeds are used in India and elsewhere as a coffee substitute. The seeds are used to extract a yellow dye.

Opera singers have for centuries used fenugreek tea for clearing excessive phlegm and mucous from the throat.

Lydia Pinkham's Vegetable Compound was widely used in the early 1900s as a remedy for various menstrual difficulties. The principal ingredient was Fenugreek, and the second Black Cohosh, with a number of minor herbs that changed with time. At its peak in 1925, the business grossed $3.8 million, enormous for the times.

Whether it worked or not is open to debate, but it is worth observing that in 1876, the year Lydia patented the formula, a prominent surgeon was urging removal of healthy ovaries to treat menstrual cramps, with a mortality rate of 40%.

A plaster for easing pain, softening swellings, and/or bringing boils to a head can be easily made by boiling an ounce each of flaxseed, marshmallow root and fenugreek seeds in milk, until thick. Spread between two cloths and apply to the affected area.

The flavour of fresh seeds is very aromatic, and somewhat reminiscent of celery and lovage. The ground seed has a very strong, maple flavour, but mealy and bitter. The aroma is like burnt sugar, but not unpleasant.

It is used to advantage in blends that imitate caramel, vanilla, butterscotch, rum and licorice; as well as unique curry powders such as vindaloo, chutneys and fish curries.

Various products such as bread, biscuits, noodles and other baked goods can contain up to 20% germinated fenugreek seed powder and still be organoleptically acceptable. Hooda & Jood, *Plant Foods Hum Nutr* 2004 59:4.

The seeds are a useful anti-oxidant for preserving foods. One study found the potential anti-oxidant effect equal to BHA and BHT. Work by Mansour et al, found beef patties from fresh and frozen meat preserved well with the seed extract. *Food Chem* 2000 69:2.

Sprouted seeds are one of our tallest and greenest sprouts. It is slightly bitter, and best combined with clover and alfalfa in a mixture. It matures in 8-9 days and does best at temperatures below 75° F.

The seed husks are an industrial source of mucilage, used to give a finish to certain fabrics in the textile industry.

The fresh and dried leaves are prized additions to East Indian cuisine. The dried leaves, from a special variety of fenugreek called **KASOORI METHI** is used in Indian cooking to enhance the flavour of tandoori sauces and gravies. The fresh leaves are cooked as a vegetable curry, turning from bitter when raw, to almost sweet.

Fresh Fenugreek leaves are extremely rich in Vitamin C (207mg%); while the dried leaves are over 32.6% crude protein.

In India, the leaves are considered aperient, and used to relieve indigestion and bilious conditions. A paste of the leaves is applied to swellings, burns, and as a hair tonic.

The seeds are considered heating and will aggravate Pitta conditions in excess.

The tops before flowering are infused for migraines.

Fenugreek also restores nitrogen to the soil, making it a useful rotation crop and forage crop with quality that matches or exceeds alfalfa.

Seed yields of 14000 kilos per hectare can be expected, based on a broadcast of 35 kg/ha of seed.

The seed is sometimes slow to germinate, and for small plots, soaking overnight in warm water will speed this up. Otherwise, waiting until the soil warms up to 50° F is another option.

Ironically, the application of nitrogen and phosphorus fertilizers increases the level of diosgenin in seeds.

Since antiquity, fenugreek seed has been valued as a medicinal fodder for livestock, helping improve their appetite. It can be used as a green mature in orchard settings, or in crop rotation.

Work by Acharya et al, at Agriculture Canada's Lethbridge Research Centre, resulted in a new form of fenugreek for forage.

Rashwan et al, *Egyptian J of Rabbit Science* 1999 8:2 found that anise, fenugreek and caraway supplementation increased feed efficiency, litter gain weight and pre-weaning mortality rates. The study supplemented only 12 grams per kilogram of weight for the does.

In India, the seeds are utilized in the manufacture of nutritional supplements for horses and cattle. The seeds are given to ruminants and chickens suffering diarrhea.

Several studies confirm the anti-oxidant potential of fenugreek seed for preserving foods.

Work by McCarthy et al, *Meat Science* 2001, 57:2 found seed extracts compared favorably with synthetic BHA and BHT, in fresh and previously frozen pork patties.

A freeze-dried extract of Fenugreek was reported to be anti-oxidant in a carotene and linoleic acid emulsion, with activity similar to commercial preservatives. Rao et al, *Nutrition Res* 1996 16.

A study in *Food Chemistry* 1998 63:1 suggests that the distribution of diosgenin changes in the plant during growth.

Ortuno et al, at the University of Murcia, Spain, looked at fenugreek plants from 15 to 60 days. Young leaves contained the highest levels at 20 mg/gram dry weight.

When they applied benzyl aminopurine at 20 ppm a 27% increase occurred after thirty days.

Work by Taylor et al, at the AgriFood station in Lethbridge found the cultivar Amber gave yields of 0.54%. Like Ortuno, they found foliage levels of diosgenin changed from 0.16 at nine weeks to 0.07 at 15 and 19 weeks.

Both Amber and Quatro varieties were developed at the University of Saskatchewan Crop Development Centre.

Brenac et al, *Phytochemistry* 1996 41:2 found steroidal sapogenins, including disogenin, accumulate rapidly in seeds 60 days after full bloom, and then decrease slightly in mature seeds.

This is good news, as the prairie climate may not always allow fully mature seed to form.

Cercospora leaf spot, a fungus, is a potential serious problem for growers in Western Canada.

Fenugreek's cousin, Blue Clover (*T. caerulea*) was grown in New World German gardens to flavour Sapsago cheese, very popular in its time.

MEDICINAL

CONSTITUENTS- seed-protein (23-30%), especially tryptophan and lysine, lipids (7%), sterols, fibre (cellulose, hemicellulose) and 25-45% soluble galactomannans (galactose mannose ratio 3:2, saponins including diosgenin (0.2-0.4%) and yamogenin, tigogenin, neotigogenin, fenugreekine, smilagenin, gitogenin, sarsasapogenin, trigofoeno-sides, and other steroidal saponin glycosides of the furostanol and spirostanol type; flavonoids including iso-orientin, vanillin, isovitexin, vitexin-7-glucoside, orientin, sapona-retin, gentianin, carpaine and vicenin-1; 4-hydroxyisoleucine, 0.13% trigonelline (coffearin, N-methylbetaine of the nicotinic acid); L-histidine, sotolone, B12 and volatile oils. Also contain 3.9-4.3% glutamic acid, arginine (2.2-2.7%), and up to 28% mucilage.
leaves and stems- diosgenin, scopoletin and gamma schizandrin, choline (1.3%), calcium (1.3%), beta carotene, d-mannose, coumarin, rutin, protopectin, myoinositol, lignan (28%), yamogenin tetrosides, vitexin, vicenins, trigoforin, fenugreekine.

The seeds are carminative, tonic and astringent, useful in diarrhea and dysentery. A neuromuscular stimulant, the seed is especially recommended for emaciated types, including diabetics, and for those suffering poor nutrition, anemia, frigidity and impotence.

The warm, dry, bitter taste of ground seeds can help stimulate and improve weakened digestion.

It will help weight gain by improving digestive absorption, and clearing of mucous from the intestine.

Consuming the seeds appears to reduce dietary fat consumption. In a double-blind, randomized, placebo-controlled, crossover study of 12 men, ingestion of seed at two different levels reduced lipid intake. Chevassus et al, *Eur J Clin Pharmacol* 2009 Oct 7.

The seeds contain mucilage that helps create bulking action in cases of constipation, but only when taken with large amounts of water. Not only does fenugreek help one gain weight, but it also helps improve protein utilization, inhibit phosphorus secretion and increase erythrocyte count.

As well, fenugreek seeds act as a lymphatic detergent. They are used in the treatment of sore throats, bronchitis, and chronic coughs with thick, and hard to remove mucous. Inflammation of the stomach, and intestine also respond to the soothing and healing properties of fenugreek. The seeds are said to be equal to quinine in preventing fevers.

Externally, the seeds also act as an emollient, softening skin and controlling skin inflammation. For this purpose they are ground and used as a poultice on the affected area. They are especially useful in cellulitis, staph infections and boils.

Work by Kawabata et al, *Planta Medica* 2011 77:7 found steroidal saponin glycosides from seeds to possess both anti-inflammatory and anti-melanogenic properties.

The seeds possess oxytocic properties, stimulating to the uterus.

Fenugreek seed was traditionally recommended to help increase breast milk and breast size; and is used today in veterinary medicine to increase milk production. Fenugreek seed can both help increase breast milk production, and eliminate or minimize vaginal dryness. In South America, the seeds are boiled in milk for this purpose.

A trial of 66 women given fenugreek, control or placebo found milk volume and weight regain of infant significantly higher in the herbal group. Turkyilmaz et al, *The J Alt Compl Med* 2011 17:2.

At the same time, however, the seed inhibits induced breast cancer in rat studies by Amin et al, *Cell Biol Int* 2005 29:8. This suggests chemo-preventative effects against breast cancers.

Khoja et al, *Asian Pac J Cancer Prev* 2011 2:12 found the seeds induce apoptosis of MCF-7 breast cancer cell lines. The seed extract induces cell death in human T lymphoma Jurkat cells, via apoptosis and autophagy. Al-Daghri et al, *BMC Compl Altern Med* 2012 Oct 30 12:202.

In Ayurvedic medicine, **METHIKÃ** is considered wholesome and laxative, and alleviator of all three doshas.

In India, the powdered seeds are considered an effective substitute for cod liver oil, and used for scrofula, anemia, gout, diabetes and debility.

The seeds are known for their anti-diabetic, blood cholesterol, and blood lipid lowering properties. Several studies in the 1980s; Ribes et al, in the *Annals of Nutrition and Metabolism* and Valette et al, *Atherosclerosis* pointed the way in this regard.

Whether this is due to the mucilage, fibre or steroidal saponins- or all three, time and more research will tell.

Research by Petit et al, *Steroids* 1995 seems to indicate the latter.

More than 100 scientific studies (mainly animal) have shown blood sugar modulation.

Fenugreek appears effective in Type 1 (child onset) diabetes. In the European Journal of Clinical Nutrition 1990, two groups of children were fed the same diets for one day. One group had 50 grams of de-bittered seed sprinkled on their lunch and dinner. This group had 54% less glucose in their urine at the end of day, and total cholesterol had been reduced, without affecting HDL, the good cholesterol.

In 2003, Sharma conducted a study giving 100 grams of de-bittered fenugreek powder for 20 days, with a 42% decrease in the ratio of HDL to LDL and VLDL.

One 1996 study from India, involved type II diabetics that took 25 grams of fenugreek for 24 weeks. It lowered their cholesterol by 14%, and triglycerides by 15%. In this crossover, placebo-controlled trial of 60 type 2 diabetic patients, the ingestion of 12.5 mg fenugreek powder twice daily in food for six months caused a 40.6% reduction in blood glucose curve.

Work by Mohammad et al, *Can J Physio Pharm* 2006 84:6 found fenugreek seed markedly decreased blood sugar levels and corrected GLUT4 in skeletal muscles.

Blood sugar reductions have been noted in numerous human clinical studies including improving peripheral glucose usage.

Daily ingestion of 25 grams of seeds for 21 days has been shown to decrease glucose in blood and urine. *Zhong Yao Xue* 1987 812-3.

Fenugreek acts like a blood sugar adaptogen, helping raise it when too low, and lower levels in blood when too high.

Fibre and galactomannan rich fractions are believed responsible, with saponins only active on elevated blood cholesterol in some studies. No one knows for sure, so why not use the whole seed.

Galactomannan is of interest to both nutraceutical and functional food industries.

Fenugreek has 50% galactose galactomannan, and is more soluble than the widely used guar gum that is only 33% galactose.

One study found an amino acid from fenugreek seed that potentiates insulin secretion. 4-hydroxyisoleucine (4-OH-Ile), *in vitro* potentiated glucose induced insulin release from non-insulin dependent diabetic rat-isolated islets. The effect, in part, is from direct pancreatic B cell stimulation. Broca et al, *American Journal of Physiology* Oct 1999.

The presence of 4-hydroxyisoleucine is believed responsible for stimulating insulin secretion and lowering blood sugar. Sauvaire et al, 1996. This is an unusual amino acid, which increases in sprouts with age. *Phytochemistry* 1997 44:4. It's main disadvantage as a functional food ingredient is the intense bitterness.

Naturex produces an extract standardized to 2% 4-hydroxysoleucine under the name Hydroxylean.

Haeri et al, *Phytother Res* 23:1 found this compound increases insulin resistance, reduces hyperglycemia and protects liver function.

Fenugreek seed extracts are comparable to metformin when fructose is fed to animals. Kannappan et al, *Ind J Med Res* 2009 129:4.

Promilin, from Technical Sourcing Int, is a complex of bioactive amino acids, including the bitter compounds, now available for use in nutraceutical and functional food products.

One mouse study, found seed extracts decreasing T3, and increasing T4 levels in the thyroid. The application to human use is uncertain. Panda et al, *Pharmacol Res* 1999 40.

Another 1999 study in *Plant Foods for Human Nutrition* asked twenty patients to add one packet daily of either 12.5 g or 18 g of fenugreek powder to their meals for a month. Those who consumed 18 grams showed a 21% reduction in LDL, or bad cholesterol, while those taking a smaller dose still had a 17% reduction.

Research at the U of Minnesota studied 18 people with BMI over 30, dividing them into three groups. One group took 4 grams of powder, another 8 grams between meals and control group none. The middle group had a greater sense of fullness, saiety and ate 10% less calories.

French research found people taking 600 mg a day of seed extract ate 17% less fat and 12% fewer calories. *Eur J Clin Pharm.*

The presence of furostanol saponins was reported, in 1919, by Wunschendorff, a French research scientist working in Algeria. Fenugreek seeds have at least a dozen different saponins. Furostanol saponins could be used in sports nutrition, helping induce muscle mass and strength.

Unlike wild yam, the fenugreek seed contains no free sapogenins, but the precursor furostanol and spirostanol glycosides.

Dr. Roland Hardman, a pharmacist at Bath University, has spent more than ten years developing species of fenugreek that yield high amounts of diosgenin from seed. The steroid diosgenin can be converted in human body to progesterone.

Taylor et al, *J Agric Food Chem* 2002 50 looked at 10 accessions of fenugreek during two summers in three locations in western Canada.

Diosgenin levels ranged from 0.28-0.92%, with four accessions in the 0.7-0.98% range. This is the work needed to build a nutraceutical industry around this unique plant.

The compound fenugreekine is a C_{27}-steroidal sapogenin-peptide ester that upon hydrolysis gives diosgenin, yamogenin and other products.

Work by Raju et al, *Cancer Epidem Biomark Prev* 2004 13:8 found diosgenin has potential as a colon cancer preventative compound. Sur et al, *Phyto Res* 15:3 found extracts reduced tumors by 70%, suggestive of neoplastic activity.

Whatever the case, fenugreek seed has a stimulating effect on bone healing, according to *Hamdard Medicus* Oct/Dec 1998 31:4. This is interesting, since Maria Treben had suggested its use for osteomyelitis, bone growth, and atrophy of the bones for many years.

Combine one half cup of yarrow tea, taken four times daily, and into two of these add one half teaspoon of ground fenugreek seeds.

Elujoba et al, reported the yield of sapogenin from the precursor can be increased by 90%, with the aqueous acid hydrolysis time reduced to 90 minutes, if the seed was first incubated at 45° C, at pH 4, with aeration for four days.

Even this incubation period can be shortened by supplementing the seed's endogenous enszymes with Naringinase D (rhamnosidase + beta-glucosidase + pectinase from *Aspergillus niger*, commercially available for de-bittering citrus fruit peel for fruit drinks. This enzyme can even be entrapped in alginate for repeated use.

Fenugreek seeds are protective of the digestive tract, helping avoid damage caused by food or drugs. Pandian et al, *J Ethnopharm* 2002 81:3.

A flour of the seeds is made into a paste in India, and used as cosmetic and poultice to inflamed parts of the body.

In that country, the seeds are used for dropsy, heart disease, and enlargements of the liver and spleen.

Fenugreekine, a steroidal sapogenin peptide ester, promotes urine flow and decreases tension; and inhibits the replication of some viruses.

In fact, fenugreekine inhibited about 80% of *vaccinia* virus replication, confirming the long held use of the seed tea as a prophylactic for chickenpox and smallpox. This may be due, in part, to nicotinic acid, itself anti-viral and anti-parasitic.

Fenugreek seed appears to possess anti-bacterial properties. Bhatti et al, reported in *Fitoterapia* 1996 67:4 flavonoids or fixed oils may be responsible for the activity shown against both gram positive and negative bacteria.

The seed has been found in animal studies to increase activity of macrophages that engulf bacteria and viruses.

Trigonelline has been shown to significantly inhibit liver carcinoma in mice. Trigonelline, when heated or degraded yields nicotinic acid, or niacin. This may explain another mechanism for lowering blood cholesterol levels.

The seed lowers blood pressure due to seratonergic antagonism involving the 5-HT_2 receptor sub-type. Balaraman et al, *Pharm Bio* 44:8.

Trigonelline, also present in hemp seeds and yarrow herb, possesses hypoglycemic activity, again fitting with diabetic support.

Preet et al, *Mol Cell Biochem* 2005 278:1-2 found a combination of fenugreek seed powder and sodium orthovanadate, a vanadium compound, helped restore glucose balance and peripheral nerve conditions such as sciatica.

Germinated fenugreek seed powder, at 18 grams daily, was tested on 20 hypo-cholesterolemic adults for one month with significant reduction in total cholesterol and LDL levels.

Fenugreek seed sprouts possess high anti-oxidant activity and in one study suggest high anti-microbial activity against peptic ulcer linked *Helicobacter pylori*. Randhir et al, *Asia Pac J Clin Nutr* 2004 13:3.

Dialysed fenugreek seed extract appears to mediate hypoglycemic effect in part by the activation of an insulin-signaling pathway in adipocytes and liver cells. Vijayakumar et al, *Br J Pharmacol* 2005 146:1.

Protodioscin, isolated from the seed, has been shown to induce cell death and apoptosis in human leukemia HL-60 lines. Hibasami et al, *Int J Mol Med* 2003 11:1.

Sathiyamoorthy et al, *Pharm Bio* 1999 37:3 found water extracts of fenugreek plants more than 80% inhibitory against cultured melanoma cell lines.

Scientists at Johns Hopkins suggest that fenugreek seed extract can slow or stop the growth of breast, pancreatic and prostate cancer cells. Shabbeer S et al, *Cancer Biol & Therapy* 2009 8(3): 272-78.

Water extracts may prevent urinary toxicity associated with cyclophosphamide. Bhatia et al, *Food Chem Tox* 44:10.

Tinnitus, or ringing in the ears, can be relieved in cases involving catarrhal deafness, or congestion of the mastoid region.

Traditional Chinese Medicine uses both roasted and unroasted seed for abdominal pains, hernias, kidney disorders, rheumatism, and impotence in men. The dried seed is known as **WOO LU BAR** or **HU LU BA** and used to lower cholesterol levels and support liver and kidney function. The Japanese call it **KOROHA**, and the Koreans, **HOROP'A**.

It clears cold and dampness from the lower abdomen and reproductive systems, and is used for leg heaviness, and dysmenorrhea with coldness in the lower abdomen and uterus. Today, pessaries of fenugreek are used in China to treat cervical cancer. In men, it helps relieve chronic prostatitis and lumbar pain. It is used mainly for Yang deficient conditions, particularly of the Kidney.

A MTH water-soluble fraction of the seeds appears to possess analgesic and anti-inflammatory properties comparable to dicolfenac sodium and other drugs. Vyas et al, *Acta Pol Pharm* 2008 65:4.

The seeds appear to reduce immune response to skin irritation in mice studies, suggesting a reduced reaction. Ali F et al, *J Comp Integr Med* 2010 7:1.

The seed is salt mix-fried to bring out the bitter and warming nature, for use in impotence, premature ejaculation due to kidney yang deficiency.

This form is also used for inguinal hernia and internal cold conditions affecting the testicles and scrotum; or dysmenorrhea and headaches associated with the same kidney yang conditions.

Tinnitus is helped in some cases, and chronic catarrhal deafness will sometimes respond to the seed combined with fresh plantain and nettle juice.

Ayurvedic medicine regards fenugreek as a sexual rejuvenator and aphrodisiac. They use the seed for digestive and bronchial complaints, allergies, neurasthenia, gout and arthritis.

A 4% seed extract ointment has been shown in six-week human clinical trials to reduce skin melanin and erythema. Wagas et al, *Acta Pol Pharm* 67:2.

The seed tea may have some benefit in preventing calcium oxalate stone formation, according to studies conducted by Ahsan et al, *Journal of Ethnopharmacology* 1989. Laroubi et al, *Phyto Res* 2007 21:10 found the seed prevents kidney calculi and urolithiasis by 27%.

The seeds are a fairly rich source of the amino acid L-histidine that shows some benefit in chronic kidney failure.

Gallstone formation and preventing its recurrence, may be helped by the seed. In an animal study in India, both high and low dose supplementation, reduced gallstones by 64% and 61% respectively, in relation to control group with no change.

Companies such as Emerald Seed Products in Saskatchewan are leading the way as a processor, and marketer of Fenugreek products for the cholesterol and diabetic markets. Their new product, FenuLife is a low-odour variety with high soluble fibre content.

When reduced to 85%, it is totally odorless, and tasteless, and can be taken as a dietary supplement, or functional food component. A particular variety, Canafon, is currently being cultivated on 1100 acres in Saskatchewan; with more to come.

Dr. Tapan Basu, my friend from the University of Alberta, has been investigating the dietary fibre and anti-oxidants in fenugreek as regards human consumption. He hopes to find varieties that contain compounds in sufficient quantity to justify growing the crop as a nutraceutical or functional food additive.

The seeds contain vitamin B12, or cyanocobalamin, that is needed to prevent pernicious anemia, and help those suffering from wasting diseases.

Carpaine has a sedative effect on the central nervous system. *Manual of Plant Medicinals and Their Active Constituents* 1986 177.

Water extracts of the germinated seed ameliorate hepatic and kidney toxicity induced by the pesticide Cypermethrin. Sushma et al, *Human & Exp Toxicol* 29:4.

Recent work by Acharya et al, at the Ag Food Canada Centre in Lethbridge, has found both anti-oxidant and anti-leukemic properties in fenugreek genotypes. Most impressive is apoptosis of CLL B cells.

The leaves possess cooling properties, and can be used externally and internally for swellings and burns. In India, the leaves known as methi are part of kitchen cuisine.

Javan et al, *J of Ethnopharmacology* 1997 58:2 looked at the pain relieving potential of fenugreek leaf.

Using tail flick tests in rats, they determined leaf extracts produce pain-relief through central and peripheral mechanisms, with anti-nociceptive effect at 2000 mg/kg, more potent than sodium salicylate at 300 mg/kg.

A follow up study in same journal 2001 75:2-3 by Ahmadiani et al, indicates unnamed alkaloids, cardiac glycosides and phenols may be responsible for the anti-inflammatory and anti-pyretic activity.

Fresh leaves are applied to the head to promote hair growth and prevent further falling of hair. Several patents for hair growth stimulating products containing trigonelline have been filed. See www.biofen.com for more info.

Pessaries can be made from the leaves and stems for treating leucorrhea.

The leaves are a good dietary source of choline, helpful in the prevention and treatment of Alzheimer's disease. The leaves are pleasant to eat and may have some application in functional foods.

Fenugreek leaf powder has been found to reduce oxidative stress in experimental diabetes. Annida et al, *J Med Food* 2005 8:3.

At one gram per kilogram of weight in diabetic rats, the leaves were similar in benefit to glibenclamide.

Abdel-Barry et al, *J Ag Food* 58:3 found water extracts of the leaf lower blood sugar in both normal and hyperglycemic animals.

Parvizpur et al, *J Ethnopharm* 104:1-2 has found the leaves possess analgesic activity, by blocking spinal purinoceptors.

Those with chickpea allergies may react to fenugreek in a similar unpleasant manner.

Fenugreek seeds are used by holistic veterinarians for arthritis in dogs.

ESSENTIAL OIL

Although the seeds are odorous, the essential oil yield is very low, at less than 0.02%. It is composed mainly of anethole; with sotoline (3-hydroxy-4, 5-dimethyl-2 (5H)-furanone), possessing the characteristic odour.

It contains up to 27% cadinene, 12% alpha cadinol, 11% gamma eudesmol, and 10.5% alpha bisabolol.

Over 50 volatile components have been detected and 39 identified. The essential oil gives a walnut like fragrance to several modern perfumes.

An oleoresin can be extracted from fenugreek seeds. Numerous volatiles including sesquiterpenoids, lactones, alkanes and furan derivatives are present. In both the steam-distilled oil from seed and from oleoresin, most components are shared with a few exceptions.

Fenugreek extract has a celery-like spiciness, with coumarin sweetness and an almost nauseating lovage-like tenacity. A little goes a long way in perfume work.

Eugenol, beta elemene, tetradecene, calarene, l-hexadecene, thymol, and camphor are present in oil from seeds, but not present in oil distilled from the oleoresin.

It is worth noting that several top notes, including undecane, 5-methyl-delta-caprolactone, dodecane, and tridecane, are present in headspace vacuum entrapment models, but not in the other two methods.

The roots were sometimes used in early Arabian perfumes.

Oil of Fenugreek is a good insect repellant.

SEED OIL

Fenugreek seed oil contains about 7% of a fixed oil, that is responsible for the odour and flavour of fenugreek. The fatty acids are mainly linoleic (60%), oleic (15%), and palmitic (12%). The very bitter taste is due to two alkaloids, trigonelline and choline.

The seed oil is considered to be a galactagogue, increasing breast milk.

The seed and oil can be made into a skin cream that is effective for erythema and reducing melanin pigmentation. Waqas et al, *Acta Pol Pharm* 2010 67:2.

HYDROSOL

Fenugreek leaf hydrosol is produced and available on the world market.

Due to the potential estrogenic effect of the young leaf stage as a medicinal herb, this floral water should be studied for potential use in hot flush sprays, and other therapies involving menopause and assorted hormone related issues.

PERSONALITY TRAITS

Fenugreek doesn't exercise much. Perhaps called lazy or even a slob, Fenugreek lives in a sedentary existence where 'exercise' becomes a dirty word, and 'work' is equally repulsive.

Fenugreek drives, but won't walk a hundred metres from the parking place to the shops. In short, there is an obvious reason why this person is a bit poddy, a bit overweight, a bit slack of muscle tone and even more obviously a little yellow in overall skin colour.

Typically they don't sweat much at all, and may seldom think of using their bladders. Fluid circulations, especially lymphatic, are slow. Strangely enough they often eat the very worst foods for their type-fatty, fast-foods, deep-fried potatoes, rich buttery sauces and then wash it all down with dry wines, or other alcohol based fluids.

Alcohol is dehydrating anyway! No wonder their livers slow down, excess fats are stored in the tissues, and it becomes harder and harder to find the energy to even think of regular exercise let alone a walk around the park with the dog.

Overweight, flabby, with an upward creeping blood pressure, through arteries narrowing from fatty plague deposition in their walls is the Negative chronic Fenugreek.

A flight of stairs can become difficult, even a downright hazard for heart and major circulation.

Handfuls of vitamins may be resorted to, or a naturopath may be consulted in a burst of guilt or with family prodding; but when exercise is advised as part of a treatment program, chronic Fenugreek loses interest. Or, even worse, in a fit of less disgust out they race in brand new jogging shoes at 5 a.m.- and drop dead three weeks later from the too-sudden major changes in circulatory pressures and fluid flows. Typically, their skin colour goes yellowish-grey after any too-sudden exercise.

The positive Fenugreek person leads a life where compulsory sitting and limited movements during working hours are balanced by regular exercise.

Positive Fenugreek goes for a brisk walk in the park in the lunch hour, or a swim before or after work. After sitting for hours in a business conference, you'll find them running upstairs two floors, not waiting for the elevator.

Graphic artists, fashion designers, authors and office workers, telephonists, machinists, even dentists, need to change their limited postural stances of the day and exercise physically to keep fluid circulations moving. Curry for dinner may also be a favourite. **HALL**

I think Fenugreek accepts the fact that, for most of its life, it is stepped upon and ignored. In the flurry of spring and summer growth, fenugreek tends to blend in with the rest of the meadow "weeds", fighting to stand out in the crowd.

But when those three or four inch seed pods begin to mature in mid to late summer, fenugreek suddenly emerges as a seasoned veteran of fields and pastures. The other plants may begin to wither and die back, but fenugreek stands out from the rest, proud to show off its impressive little fruit pods. Sometimes I can almost hear it say, "I'm little, but don't ever underestimate me." **DEWEY**

Fenugreek's keyword is realignment. Fenugreek is a powerful hormonal aligner and facilitates transition such as puberty, childbirth, menopause or mid-life crisis. Fenugreek is useful anytime when there is a real fundamental shift and hormones need to be realigned into the new pattern. **MULDERS**

BOTANICA POETICA

Let us speak of Fenugreek
Of the family of Pea
Grown in warmer climate
It's as ancient as can be
The seed is food and medicine
Around the globe it's used
In India for a curry dish
In Africa, a coffee food
It's a bitter for the appetite
For anorexia a friend
In dyspepsia and gastritis
It can heal and mend
It decreases the blood sugar
Lowers cholesterol too
Acting as a fiber
A digestive aid for you
Because it's so emollient
It can help to heal a wound
On skin with inflammation
A sore throat it can soothe
An expectorant if you're congested
It's a tonic in a seed
Demulcent and nutritive
Increase milk flow if you need
A young woman might take it
For breasts she thinks are flat
An aphrodisiac some say
You can be the judge of that!

SYLVIA CHATROUX

RECIPES

TINCTURE- 20 drops three times daily. Crushed seed 1:5 in 30% alcohol.

DECOCTION- 2 tsp crushed seed to one cup of water, infuse fve hours and then heat and simmer for one minute. Take 6-8 ounces four to six times daily.

CAPSULES- 500 mg caps 4-12 daily as needed.

FENUGREEK "MAPLE" SYRUP- Take one half-cup seeds and soak in one cup of water for eight hours. Add two ounces of honey and blend until smooth. Artifical maple syrup uses corn syrup, probably GMO corn. Avoid

ORIGINAL LYDIA PINKHAM'S VEGETABLE COMPOUND- Four parts fenugreek seeds, three parts True Unicorn root (*Aletris farinosa*), two parts each, of Black Cohosh, Pleurisy Root and Life Root (*Senecio aureus*).

CAUTION- Fenugreek has some complex constituents, and may interfere with some diabetic drugs, MAO inhibitors, or blood thinning or heart medications.

The seed is contraindicated for patients with deficient yin and true heat signs. Pregnant women should be aware of the coumarin and estrogen type components of fenugreek and use caution due to oxytocic influence.

In small amounts the FDA places fenugreek as GRAS for food use.

A false diagnosis of maple syrup urine disease was reported in the New England Journal of Medicine, based on a five-week old infant drink herbal tea containing fenugreek seed. A compound in the seed, solotone is responsible for the characteristic aroma associated with the disease, caused by improper breakdown of isoleucine, leucine and valine, due to deficiency of enzymes needed to do so. Solotone builds up in body and infants die unless put on strict diet that is devoid of amino acids mentioned.

Fenugreek contains a number of potential allergenic proteins, in most cases due to cross reactivity with peanuts. In the case of patients with latter allergy, it would be best to identify another herb for use.

LANCE LEAFED FIGWORT
(*Scrophularia lanceolata* Pursh.)
KNOTTED FIGWORT
COMMON FIGWORT
(*S. nodosa* L.)
PARTS USED- leaves, flowers, roots

I will pluck the figwort,
With the fruitage of sea and land,
The plant of joy and gladness,
The plant of rich milk.

SCOTTISH CHARM

Scrophularia derives from the use of the plant for throat infections including scrofula (tubercular swellings of the neck's lymph nodes) and swollen lumps. Hence, one of the older names, throat wort. Scrofula may derive from the Latin **STRUO** meaning to build up, referring to a swelling or tumor.

Hemorrhoids were known colloquially as figs; and to the Romans **FICUS** meant both the condition and the fruit. In medieval medicine hemorrhoids, required the application of the root of figwort, which has fig-like knobs. Ficus also referred to head scabs under the hair.

The German botanist, Otto Brunfels, named the plant Figwort in 1623.

Although introduced to the prairies, figwort is a common plant in isolated patches. Its leaves and stems have a putrid smell, similar to Elder leaves, when crushed, only rivaled by the foul acrid scent of the root; both lost in drying. Lance leafed Figwort is native to western North America.

Figwort is one of the few plants in nature that bears greenish-purple, brown flowers that smell like human sweat combined with honey. This helps attract wasps for nectar breaks, and spread pollen.

It was hung around the home for its protective powers, or around the neck to help keep the wearer healthy, attract good fairies and protect against evil spirits.

The Iroquois used decoctions of the root for hemorrhage after childbirth, or in prevention of colds and cramping after giving birth. Leaf poultices were applied to sunburns, sunstroke and frostbite. The herb was added to mixtures for water retention.

The Welsh call it **DEILEN DDU** or good leaf; while in Ireland, it is regarded as the Queen of Herbs, and consort of Foxglove. The Gaelic name **FOTHROM** is a corruption of **FAOI TROM**, meaning under the elder.

Its bitter taste was put to use in making ales. The Irish used *S. nodosa* ointment for "burnt holes", or gangrenous chicken pox.

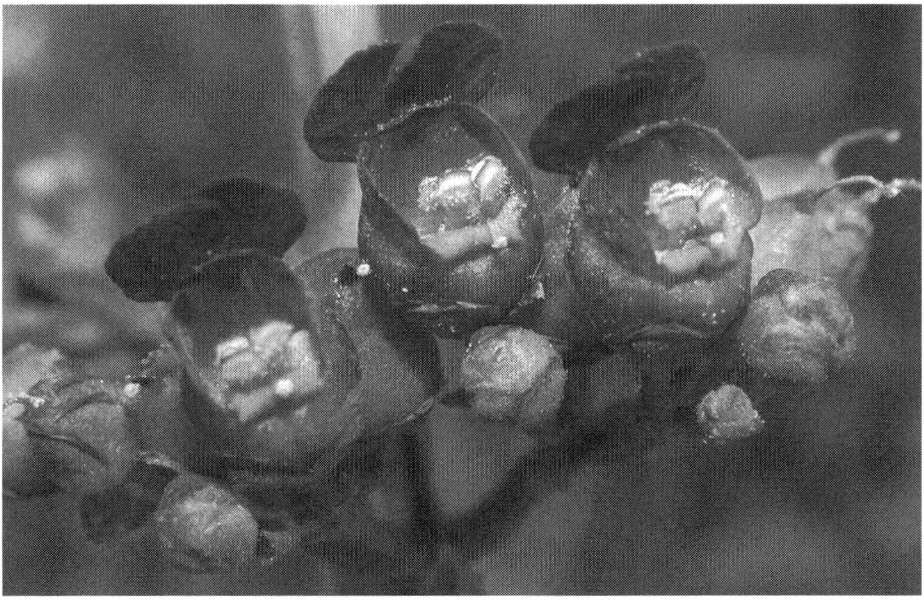

Common Figwort flowers

Eclectic physicians used it in Compound Scrophularia syrup, a mixture used for cancer that has moved into the lymphatic system. Dr. Ellingwood described the plant picture of the patient as having marked evidence of cachexia, toxic blood, and puffiness in the face with full, pallid lips.

Eli Jones suggested it is "one of the most valuable remedies we have in the treatment of cancer in its advanced stages, when there are lumps in the neck and in the axilla."

In Japanese Kampo medicine, the related *S. ningpoensis*, is called **GENJIN**, and used for the softening and dissipating of lymphatic nodules like the Western tradition.

The Chinese use the same figwort. Experiments in that country indicate figwort can cool the blood, bring down blood pressure and reduce blood sugar. Known as **XUAN SHEN** it is used for sadness, swellings and pain of the throat, constipation and painful urination. It is prepared in salt for fluid imbalances.

For some unknown reason, the plant is very attractive to wasps. Other than that, it is a very good pesticide, and can be cold infused and macerated at 5% to spray on affected plants.

MEDICINAL

CONSTITUENTS- *S. lanceolata* plant- steroptene, propionic, cinnamic, acetic and butyric acids, lecithin, saponins, diosmin, hesperidin, aucubin, cardioactive glycosides, haragophytum iridoids, pectins, and phenolic acids. Also contains dulcitol, galactitol, euonymit, melanpyrite, melampyrum, melampyrin.
S. nodosa- similar structure, with the addition of 18 acylated iridoid glycosides and 9 phenylethanoid glycosides in the aerial parts. Flavonoids include diosmetin, diosmin, acacetin rhamnoside, rhein; iridoids include aucubin, acetyl harpagide, harpagide, harpagoside, isoharpagoside, procumbid, and 6 alpha-rhamnopyranosyl catalpol. Phenolics include ferulic, isoferulic, p-coumaric, caffeic, cinnamic, vanillic, syringic and chlorogenic acids; present as both esters and glycosides. Also scrophulasaponins I-IV, scropoliosides, scopolioside, and stachyose.
Amino acids include alanine, isoleucine, leucine, lysine, phenylalanine, threonine, tyrosine and valine.
Harpagide is found in plant, harpagosides in root.

A fresh leaf or root tincture or strong tea can be applied to all forms of fungal infections of the skin. This includes dermatitis, cradle cap, ringworm and athlete's foot. The fresh plant can also be made into a soothing salve (see below), or a fresh poultice of leaves for diaper rashes, vaginal irritations, blocked milk duct, etc.

Figwort root is a mild stimulant of the hepatic system and general blood purifier. It is also a cleanser of the lymphatic system; especially useful for swollen glands, chronic tonsillitis, tonsil hypertony, lymph edema, lipoma, hemorrhoids and cystic breasts, The herb combines well with red clover, violet, burdock or self heal depending upon the particular constitution.

Use with red root and cleavers for hemorrhoids and general lymphatic congestion.

Combine with yellow dock root for obstinate constipation associated with damp heat.

For appendicitis, is combines well with echinacea and dandelion root; while for goitre, it combines well with cleavers as a gargle not swallowed. In Waterford, Ireland, an ointment is rubbed into the enlarged thyroid gland.

A famous Dr. Scudder Alternative formula combines figwort (*S. nodosa*), yellow dock root, alder bark, corydalis root and violet.

Lance-leaved Figwort is a mildly laxative, bitter tonic in cases of constipation and hemorrhoids. The dried plant tea is good for hives, back and chest eruptions and as a general cleanser.

It combines well with the docks for eczema, with redness and itching, and for frequent sore throats and cold sores.

Figwort helps reduce body temperature and blood pressure when used internally, in small doses. It is a mild sedative.

Figwort washes, fomentations and compresses help to reduce suppurative swellings or sprains, as well as lesions of the skin, orchitis, mastitis and lymphadenitis. Various fungal and parasitic skin infections such as tinea, ringworm, scabies and lice are likewise relieved with repeated applications. This is due in part to rhein, an anti-fungal agent also found in *Rumex* roots.

Michael Moore adds. "Figwort is a subtle and useful long-term anti-inflammatory for people with chronic, low-grade skin and mucosa sores and irritations. If you get frequent cold sores or rectal aches and have a tendency for sore throat, or if you have a long-standing eczema with periodic acute episodes of redness and itching, try this plant with some Yellow Dock in the evening…The salve or a poultice, applied laterally from armpit to nipple, helps decrease occasional PMS breast pain…

For the slow viruses (CFS, CMV, EBV and HIV) with a tendency to somewhat enlarged lymph nodes, try Figwort with Redroot mornings and evenings until the swelling decreases, then use only as an evening dose. This isn't for the infection itself but to lessen the distal lymph node congestion."

Scrofula refers to a swelling of cervical glands associated with tuberculosis, particularly bovine TB. Cervical tuberculosis occurs more often than one thinks, and is more than simply enlarged lymph nodes.

Anny Schneider suggests inserting a rolled-up figwort leaf into the vagina, petiole out, for treating vaginitis. Do this nightly, remove in morning and repeat for ten evenings.

Figwort has a mild, sedative effect, soothing the mind as well as physical irritations. It combines well with Devil's Club or Bogbean for arthritis, gout and edema aggravated by cold and wet weather. Aucubin is mildly laxative, and increases the excretion of uric acid, as does harpagoside. Figwort has the same qualitative iridoid composition as Devil's Claw, but half the content of harpagoside, explaining in part the cardiotonic and anti-inflammatory properties. It is a suitable substitute for arthritic conditions.

In France, figwort claims indication of use identical to Devil's Claw.

Recent work has found a level of harpagoside in the leaves of *S. nodosa,* similar to the roots of Devil's Claw. This makes a fresh leaf tincture useful for functional and arthritic joint disease and may be of particular benefit in psoriatic arthritis. Gordon et al, *J Am Acad Derm* 2006 54.

Graeme Tobyn and Allison Denham in their excellent text *The Western Herbal Tradition*, suggest figwort for patients vulnerable to eczema caused by bacterial infections and in diabetics subject to poor wound healing and chronic skin conditions. They suggest its use for psoriatic arthritis and lymphadenitis as well as inflamed and swollen hemorrhoids.

Rhein is laxative, with anti-fungal activity and ferulic acid has been shown to possess cholagogue properties.

Figwort and boneset leaf decoctions can be made into a suitable cough syrup with the addition of honey.

For lymphatic congestion associated with low-grade viral infections like chronic fatigue, Epstein-Barr, or HIV, it combines with cleavers and lomatium. Dr. Boericke suggested figwort for treating Hodgkin's

Disease, or lymphadenoma. It combines well with licorice root and echinacea to resolve the accompanied skin itching.

Eclectic symptoms for figwort include full and pale lips, and skin that is puffy, edematous and peculiar pink color.

Dr. Blakely proved the herb in 1866, and gave 20 drops of the tincture in repeated doses. This caused fullness of head and vertigo, bleeding of the gums, salivation, increased appetite, colic, general weariness and sleepiness, with sallow skin. Activity appeared directed towards the liver in this particular case.

Figwort root has mild pancreatic stimulating abilities, and is useful in combinations for mild diabetic tendency. It may, however, interfere with insulin uptake, so caution is advised.

Scientific studies have shown figwort to have strong antibiotic effect, especially against *Pseudomonas aeruginosa*.

Figwort (*S. nodosa*) dried seed pods contain three acylated iridoid glycosides shown to stimulate the growth of human dermal fibroblasts. This explains, in part, the traditional use of the plant for healing wounds. Stevenson et al, *Phytother Res* 2002 15:9.

The same author found scrophuroside anti-inflammatory, and scopolioside to be immune stimulating as well.

Work by Garg et al, *Phytother Res* 1994 8 and Rios et al, *Planta Med* 1991 57 (suppl 2) also identified fibroblast wound healing activity.

The root decoction removes retained placenta, and relieves pain during difficult, delayed, clotty or painful menstruation.

Infusions of *S. nodosa* on sedated rabbits, cats and dogs showed considerable reduction of arterial pressure, stimulated respiration, and lengthened PQ segment (the interval between atrial and ventricle contraction). It also changed the configuration of the T wave, which represents re-polarization of the ventricles on an ECG. The herb increased the amplitude and slowed down the frequency of contractions on isolated frog heart. Work by Karimova et al, 1996 suggests saponins at work, but nothing for certain. This work showed infusions inhibit locomotor activity and prolonged sleep in lab animals.

Harpagide shows anti-protozoal activity at an IC_{50} of 2 microg/ml. Tasdemir et al, *Phytomed* 2008 15:3.

The aerial parts of the related *S. frutescens* has been examined for cytostatic activity against Hep-2 cells derived from human carcinoma of the larynx, and McCoy cells, derived from the synovial fluid in the knee joint of a patient suffering from degenerative arthritis. High activity was noted, especially in the cinnamic group compounds.

Work by Galindez et al, *Pharm Biology* 2002 40:1 reviews the biological activity from numerous members of the genus.

HOMEOPATHY

Knotted Figwort (*S. nodosa*)

This is a valuable, powerful, slow-acting medicine in cases of enlarged lymphatic glands, including Hodgkin's disease, and lymphosarcoma.

It is a valuable skin remedy, with special affinity for dissipation of breast tumours, cystic breasts and other lumpy tissue. Cradle cap is relieved in a child.

It relieves vaginal itching, eczema about and behind the ear, and painful hemorrhoids.

Vertigo is made worse by standing, with sore eyeballs and spots before the eyes.

Pain in the sigmoid flexure, and rectum inflammation are likewise helped.

The skin on the back of the hand may be prickly and itchy. Skin rash from nickel allergy.

Ailments from suppressed anger, dreams of blood and bleeding.

The patient may be very drowsy in the morning as well as before and after meals. All symptoms are worse from lying on the right side.

DOSE- Tincture and first potency. Apply locally to cancerous glands. The mother tincture is prepared from the fresh plant before flowering. Self-experimentation by Franz, clinical observations by Cooper, Boericke and Mangialavori.

ROOT OIL

Sun infused oil of figwort is later made into salves for mastitis, hemorrhoids, and numerous other skin complaints. Best results are from the fresh roots, spring or fall, crushed in oil (1:5) and shaken daily for ten days. In cool climates use crockpot.

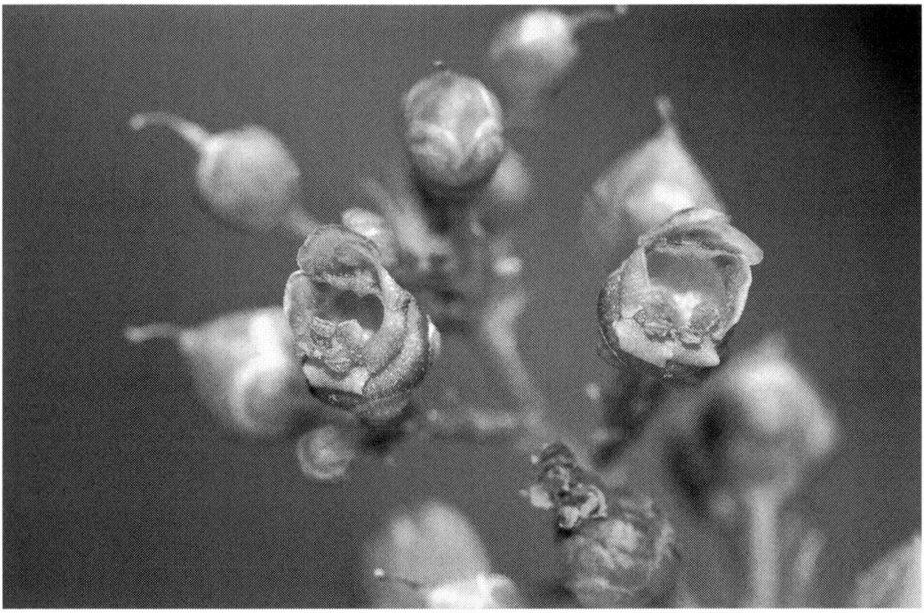

Figwort flowers

HYDROSOL

The distilled water of the whole plant, roots and all...dries up the superfluous, virulent moisture of hollow and corroding ulcers; it takes away all redness, spots, and freckles in the face, as also the scruf, and any foul deformity therein. **CULPEPPER**

Figwort water is distilled from the root and leaves, and is good for piles and faces that appear leprous. **BRUNSCHWIG**

FLOWER ESSENCES

Figwort flower essence is for agitation, anxiety, nasty dispositions, and general fear when someone is jumpy. **PEGASUS**

Figwort is for overcoming judgment towards matter. For those who love material existence and see it as a vehicle for spirit. **HABUNDIA**

Figwort flower essence keeps perspective on sense of duty, and responsibility for general public. It helps provide position in the cosmic whole. **MIRIANA**

SPIRITUAL PROPERTIES

Figwort itself is associated with shady streams and riverbanks, undergrowth and forest ditches. He [Pelikan] observes the strong rootstock with tubers arising from nodes, and how, though the panicle rises and separates from the banked pairs of nettle-like leaves—these nettle-like leaves plus the throaty flowers suggesting strongly the Lamiaceae—does not lead to the light, but to a dull brown olive-green gullet 'smelling as gloomy as nightshade' and speaking of the forces of the dark working in them. **TOBYN**

Figwort awakens the crown chakra, so that the individual will be drawn almost unconsciously to various people. It can enhance relationships on the purely spiritual level.

There is a cleansing action as well. This is partly seen in the signature, the purplish coloration.

There is a tendency for the plant to retain moisture in the most unique way. For individuals, this means that the emotional body can be viewed and understood more easily when taking the herb. They can see its purpose from a spiritual perspective; partners in relationship could take together.

The ability to love, in spite of fighting and difficulties is sometimes based on the psychic intuition that what lies ahead is worth the trouble. This may be because an individual is likely to learn and grow if willing.

Figwort's karmic purpose is to enhance relationships. When Venus and Uranus interact, this is a good time for figwort. **GURUDAS**

PERSONALITY TRAITS

Herein lies the dilemma for Scrophulariaceae. On the one hand there is the fearful, withdrawn, closed-in state necessary to be protected from injury. On the other hand there is the tranquilized, calm and relaxed state allowing joy and carefree sociability. However, in order to completely suppress all fear and anger, sedation can go too far by creating vulnerable somnolence. Then it is time to arouse the fears leading to the unpalatable, morose withdrawal for protection.

VERMEULEN

In former days this herb was relied on for the cure for toothache, and for expelling the particular disembodied spirit, or "mare", which visited our Saxon ancestors during their sleep after supper, being familiarly known to them as the "nightmare".

The "Echo" was in like manner thought by the Saxons to be due to a spectre, or mare, which they called the "wood mare".

DOCTRINE OF SIGNATURES

The doctrine of signatures suggests the plant is good for skin problems, due to the glandular nodes found on the root and leaves. In fact, the root looks so much like the connected lymph nodes of the body it is hard to miss.

It also happens to be true. Many farmers use decoctions of the fresh plant for scab and other skin problems on hogs.

However, as Michael Moore points out- "Figwort could just as easily, by that doctrine, have been used for the following.

Mouth problems (shape of flowers), heart disease (shape of leaves), cut and abrasions (leaf serrations), or ligament problems (form of stem), not to mention clotting of blood (colour of the flowers)."

Matthew Wood continues. "putrefacation (smell of flowers), swollen glands and hemorrhoids (nodular seed capsules), and fistulous discharges of pus (shape of roots). In fact, *Scrophularia* is used for all these complaints.

What is necessary for the appropriate use of the doctrine of signatures is a sense of the underlying pattern in the plant that emerges out through its signatures." **WOOD**

BOTANICA POETICA
Cleaning from the inside out
Here's an herb to use
Diuretic, purgative
And tonifying too
Ultimately helps the skin
Achieve a finer glow
Eczema and psoriasis
Itching, off you go!
Help the body function well
Soothe an inflammation
Flowers, leaves and shoots
Help rectal irritation
Not to use in pregnancy
Or if the heart is ticking wrong
But in the matters of the skin
Figwort is standing strong.
SYLVIA CHATROUX MD

RECIPES

LEAF INFUSION- One tsp dried herb to pint of boiling water. Two to 4 ounces daily.

TINCTURE-10-40 drops 3X daily of dried root 1:5, 45% alcohol tincture. For fresh whole plant tincture 1:2 at 60%. Take 30-60 drops three times daily for joint inflammation and pain. Pick the whole plant, including root before flower.

FLUID EXTRACT- 30-60 drops daily

ROOT DECOCTION- Simmer 2-4 grams of dried root to 8 oz of water fifteen minutes. Steep for one hour more. Take one ounce three times daily.

SALVE- Mash the fresh plant and immerse in four times olive or canola oil for two weeks. Shake daily. Strain and warm. Add enough beeswax to make firm ointment on cooling. Stir while cooling to ensure even dispersal.

CAUTION- Michael Moore suggested use of figwort be avoided during pregnancy, lactation and by those with heart tachycardia, on a pacemaker, or taking heart medication.

It is related to foxglove, and does contain cardiac glycosides, but in small amounts.

It should be avoided by those with hypoglycemia, colitis or diarrhea.

FORSYTHIA
KOREAN GOLDENBELLS
KOREAN FORSYTHIA
EARLY FORSYTHIA
(*Forsythia ovata* [Nakai] Vahl**)**
WEEPING FORSYTHIA
GOLDENBELLS
(*F. suspensa* [Thunb.] Vahl.**)**
GREEN STEM FORSYTHIA
(*F. viridissima* Lindley**)**
BORDER FORSYTHIA
(*F. x intermedia*)
WHITE FORSYTHIA
(*Abeliophyllum distichum* Nakai**)**
PARTS USED- flowers, leaves, berry, calyx

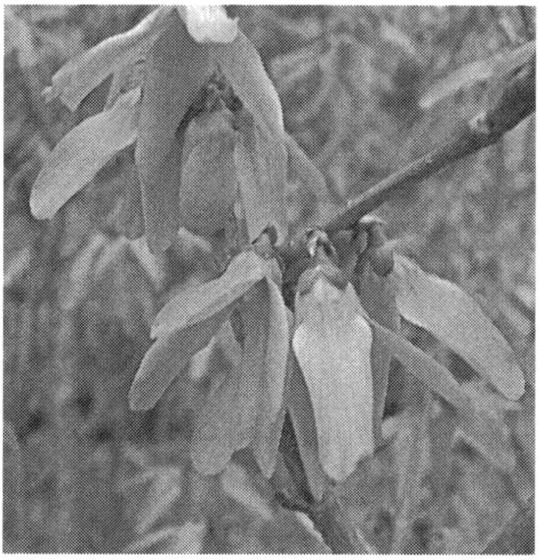

Border Forsythia

Forsythia is named in honour of William Forsyth, an 18th century horticulturist and botanist at England's Royal Gardens at Kensington and St. James. In some ways, this is quite unfortunate, as they should have an oriental name after their origin. Forsyth wrote several horticultural books, including *Treatise on the Cultivation and Management of Fruit Trees*. Suspensa means hanging, in reference to the dangling golden blooms.

Forsythia is a genus of the olive family, and at one time was known as *Ligustrum suspensum*, and placed with the privets.

The Danish botanist, Martin Vohl gave the present binomial name in 1804.

Korean Forsythia is reported in some texts to be hardy only to zone 5, and yet it grows well in protected areas of the prairie. The better-known medicinal species, Weeping Forsythia, is said to be hardy to zone 4 in the same texts, so should do well in this climate. Hardiness of -32 to -34° C is noted. I see it in front yards all over Edmonton.

Both are prone to winter kill when snow cover is inadequate. The shrub grows best in a sunny exposure with shelter from the wind. The hybrid *intermedia* is slightly more winter hardy.

The bright yellow flowers arrive early in spring, and are followed by seed capsules. All three species may be used in medicine, and are interchangeable.

If you cut lengthwise in a twig of *suspensa* species you will notice it solid at the nodes, but hollow between, while species *viridissima* is chambered throughout.

The fresh flowers and leaves can be dried and used as a pleasant herbal infusion.

The fruit has long been used in China for medicinal purpose. It was first mentioned in Shen Nong Ben Cao Jing, a manuscript written in the 1st century AD.

The plants can be started from seed, root division, cuttings or layering. When using seed, best results will be obtained from stratifying for about two months in damp sand. The seeds should be barely covered with soil, and kept moist until germination and emergence. Cuttings are best done in spring, by cutting on the node itself, which will quickly develop roots.

The green forsythia fruits, known as **QING LIAN QIAO** in Traditional Chinese Medicine, are harvested in early September, while still unripe. They are parboiled or steamed for short time and then dried in the sun, or in a commercial dryer at low temperature.

The yellow, or old seeds, known as **LIAN QIAO**, are vine ripened and harvested in late September. The seeds were traditionally removed and the capsules dried for medicinal purpose. The seeds are rich in active chemical compounds and are now considered part of the herbal product.

The fruit is also known as **ERH TS'AO**, meaning Ear Grass, **YI QIAO**, Strange Beauty, **JIAN HUA**, Orchid Flower, **SHE GEN**, Broken Root, and **SAN LIAN**, meaning Three Honesties.

In Japanese Kampo Medicine, the fruit is known as **RENGYO**, with the green half-ripe fruit considered the best.

A row of shrubs should be planted no closer than five feet apart.

Forsythia suspensa extracts reduced oxidative stress and improved broiler chicken growth under 32° C temperatures. Wang et al, *Poultry Sci* 2008 87:7.

Border Forsythia, is a sterile hybrid, and does not set fruit.

The leaves and seeds contain (-)-arctigenin, a compound found in burdock.

White Forsythia (*A. distichum*) is not a true forsythia, but in a totally different genus.

The plant scent is exquisite, similar to neroli, or orange blossoms. It is hardy to minus 34° Celsius.

MEDICINAL

CONSTITUENTS- fruit- *F. suspensa*- various triterpenoid saponins including forsythin (phillyrin); forsythol, forsythoside A (3.84%), cornoside, bigelovin, dihydrobeigelovin, rengyosides A-C, salidroside, rengyol, rengyoxide, rengyolone, suspensaside, philligenin, (+)-pinoresinol 0-beta-D- glucoside, arctiin, arctigenin, forsythine, sterols, taraxasteryl palmitate, iridoid alkaloids, flavonoids, coumarins, lignans; oleanolic, ursolic and betulinic acids; matairesinoids.
leaves- contain four lignans, four lignan glycosides, rutin, and two caffeoyl glycosides of 3,4-dihydroxyphenethyl alcohol, as in fruit. Forsythoside A content is 7.63%.
The leaves do not contain suspensaside or beta hydroxy-aceteoside.
seeds- forsythoside A (7.46%).
Flowers- phillyrin (+)-pinoresinol-beta-D-glucoside, forsythoside A, rutin, ursolic and oleanolic acid.
flower pollen- 10% rutin
F. koreana- forsythid, forsythidmethyl ester, forsythin (phillyrin). suspensaside, beta hydroxyacetoside, forsythiaside, aceteoside.
F. viridissima- arctiin, matairesinoside, oleanolic acid, aceteoside, beta hydroxy-aceteoside.
A. distichum- fresh leaves- calceolarioside D, verbascoside, cornoside, ruint, halleridone and neocal-ceolarioside D.

Forsythia capsule or fruit valve is a cold, and detoxifying remedy, used for its anti-inflammatory, anti-microbial and immune stimulating properties.

Conditions such as influenza, and colds, as well as childhood infections like chicken pox and measles are quickly resolved.

It is especially useful in acute viral, bacterial, or fungal infections, where lymphatic congestion and accumulation of pus and poisons present.

This makes the fruit useful in breast tumours, mastitis, or subcutaneous nodules in the neck. The fruit disperses clumped blood and encourages the smooth flow of qi and blood, reducing swollen lymph nodes.

Studies have shown water extracts of the fruit to possess activity against both gram positive and negative bacteria, including *Staphylococcus aureus, Streptococcus hemolyticus, Hemophilus pertussis, Diplococcus pneumoniae, Mycobacterium tuberculosis, Pseudomonas aeruginosa, Shigella, Salmonella,* and *E. coli.*

Forsythiaside is considered the most powerful anti-bacteriostatic compound of fruit and may be considered a marker of quality.

The fruit seeds show anti-viral activity against RSV. Zhang et al, *J Herb Pharm* 2002 2:3.

Forsythiaside A, also found in leaves, is active against *Staphylococcus aureus.*

The leaves possess alpha glucosidase inhibitors, suggesting use in blood sugar elevation, by preventing sugar from intestinal absorption into bloodstream. Kang et al, *Zhongquo Zhong Yao Za Zhi* 2010 35:9.

This substance inhibits inflammation and swelling. Other studies suggest dammarane triterpenes, or caffeoyl glycosides are involved in reducing inflammation. Ozaki et al, *Biol Pharm Bull* 1997 20:861 & 2000 23:365.

Skin conditions, both short and long term, associated with fungal infections, boils, ulcers, erysipelas, erythema or any long standing stagnation, are addressed. It combines well with Dandelion leaf for external sores. One name for the fruit is **CHUANG JIA SHENG YAO**, which means "sage-like herb for sores", in reference to its ability to disperse and penetrate.

It is a similar remedy to Marigold, also a golden yellow flower, but is more draining and cooling, from an energetic perspective. Marigold is warming.

Recent work in China has shown the fruit to be quite effective in treating acute nephritis. Decoctions taken three times daily before meals, while avoiding pungent and salty foods, were found effective in 8 patients after only 5-10 days. Before treatment, all eight suffered hypertension and edema, and afterwards, six had complete reduction of edema, and the other two were much improved.

In one study of eight patients with acute nephritis, the seed decoction taken three times daily before meals, showed good results. *Jiang Xi Yi Yao* 1961 7:18.

The fruit combines well with cleavers or figwort in the treatment of lymphadenitis, and as a gargle for various throat infections. It combines well with plantain seed for dysuria.

For the initial stage of fever, headache and thirst combine with Burdock seed and Wild Mint.

Thrombocytopenic purpura and allergic purpura patients have been satisfactorily cured with seed decoctions. *Guang Dong Zhong Yi* 1960 10:469.

In Kampo medicine, the fruit is one of the most effective medicines for inflammation of the gums, throat, tongue and mouth.

Lesser known is its use as a hemostat, particularly for retinal hemorrhage, and its mild cardiac tonic effect in excess Heart Yang conditions, and control after stroke. Rutin content may play a role in preventing capillary fragility, and recurrent hemorrhage, involving the eyes, lungs, bleeding stomach ulcers, and nephritis.

It combines well with Bean seed to eliminate toxic damp heat, and therefore good for jaundice with painful urinary dribbling, as well as pelvic inflammatory disease associated with damp heat congestion.

One component of the fruit, forysythiaside, is both anti-bacterial and anti-oxidant. Qu et al, *J Pharm Pharmacol* 2008 60:2

For increased absorption of compounds, it appears that adding chitosan is helpful. Zhon et al, *Phytomedicine* 2012 20:1.

The so-called green forsythia is best for clearing heat, resolving toxins and treating fever, while yellow forsythia is better for dispersing swelling, nodulations, and skin inflammations.

Fruit lignans show significant inhibition of platelet activating factor (PAF). Iwakami et al, *Chem Pharm Bulletin* 1992 40:5.

Pinoresinol and its glycoside inhibit cyclic adenosine monophosphate phospho-diesterase. Nikaido et al, *Chem Pharm Bull* 1981 29.

One experiment with fruit involved intramuscular injections of 1 ml of the crude herb twice weekly to treat lung abscesses. Of 25 patients thus treated, 14 were completely cured, and another 10 were much improved. One patient died.

The fruit is anti-bacterial against *E. coli* and *Salmonella*, as well as bacteria associated with staph infections, tuberculosis and pneumonia.

Alcohol extracts appear to contain more analgesic and anti-inflammatory activity than water preparations.

Arctigenin, isolated from the fruit, is anti-inflammatory. Kay et al, *J Ethnopharm* 2007 Nov 26.

The stems and leaves, known as **LIAN QIAO JING YE** have been used traditionally as a decoction to treat excess heat in the heart and lungs.

The root, **LIAN QIAO GEN** is a cold, bitter, and mildly toxic medicine, used for treating fever and jaundice; as well as a circulatory stimulant.

Root decoctions have also been used to wash sores, including cancerous lesions.

The seed, called **LIAN QAIO XIN** is superior for high fever, delirium, or loss of consciousness associated with pericardium aggravation.

ESSENTIAL OILS

The leaf, seed and bark of Forsythia (*F. suspensa*) contain a variety essential oils such as gamma terpinene, alpha pinene, beta phellendrene, beta pinene, mycrene, camphene, p-cymene, beta ocimene, linalool, terpinene-4-ol, carene and nor-lapachol.

It shows a broad spectrum of activity against *Staphylococcus aureus, Diplococcus pneumoniae, Bacillus dysenteriae,* hemolytic *Streptococcus, Neisseria catarrhalis, Salmonella typhi, E. coli, Mycobacterium tuberculosis, B. proteus, Bordetella pertussis, Corynebacterium diphtheriae*, leptospirosis and various influenza viruses. *Shan Xi Xin Yi Yao* 1980 9:11 51.

FLOWER ESSENCES

Forsythia (*F. suspensa*) flower essence is the remedy for addictive mental, emotional and physical patterns- those which fill us with self-loathing and yet we feel powerless to change. It grants us the ability to find our way out of the darkness and into light.

Forsythia helps us to respond intuitively and spontaneously with what really is "right action" for use. It is a catalyst for change. **PACIFIC**

Forsythia (*F. suspensa*) brings an awareness of how we gain and lose energy. Helps us to make better use of it. Gives a better appreciation of life force. **HAREBELL**

PERSONALITY TRAITS

In England, forsythia is still used in the festival of Jack-in-the-Green. On the day of the festival the chimney sweeps dance along the streets bearing a large wicker basket in which lies an infant covered with green leaves. The basket is gay with forsythia and other spring flowers. The baby within symbolizes the spirit of the coming to life of nature, the essence of all early growing plants.

Later, in folklore, the child became the "Green Man", and still later "Robin of Wood". The next title is Robin of Spring Leaves, and finally Robin Hood. The head of this legendary hero is carved in the corbets of many old English churches with flowers springing from his head and a beard of leaves. He is the Green Knight of the May festival and Maid Marion is the Queen. **GUILLET**

DOCTRINE OF SIGNATURES

Forsythia fruit is bitter, thus cools heat. Its shape is round and pointed, empty inside with a chamber very much like the heart, thus it specifically cools heat in Heart patients. These are inherent, natural characteristics, not forced or appended sophistry.

Furthermore, all herbs which are light in weight, and empty or soft inside must have opening, draining, disseminating, and unblocking functions, thus it can also disperse clumps while draining and transforming heat in the collateral channels.

RECTIFICATION OF THE MEANING OF MATERIA MEDICA

RECIPES

INFUSION- 10-30 grams. The unripe fruit is considered the best, use dried.

TINCTURE- 2-5 ml

CAUTION- Do not use in cases of diarrhea caused by deficient spleen or stomach, in those suffering fever due to Qi deficiency, patients with ulcerated carbuncles or active cold sores. In Sweden, the herb is classified as a drug, and only available from pharmacies. Do not use during pregnancy.

CANADIAN MOONSEED
YELLOW PARILLA
VINE MAPLE

(*Menispermum canadense* L.)
(*M. angulatum* Moench.)
PARTS USED- bark

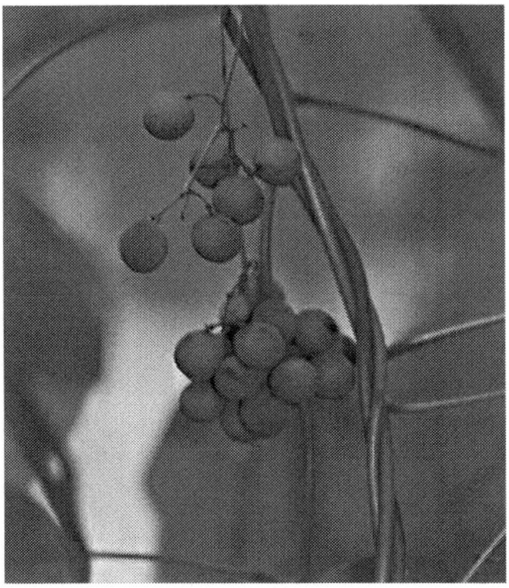

Canadian Moonseed
(Courtesy of Walter Muma)

Menispermum means Moonseed, as the seed is shaped like the crescent moon. Canadense means, of Canada. Parilla comes from its superficial appearance to the Smilax species.

Moonseed, or Yellow Parilla is of the Moonseed family, a mainly tropical grouping with 78 genera and over 500 species.

It is related to Pareira, which is used for curare, an arrow poison in South America; Calumba root, and *Cocculus indicus,* another important homeopathic plant. In fact, it is used as a bitter tonic in a manner very similar to Calumba root due in large part to its berberine content.

Our Moonseed is a vine up to three metres long, found in the woods of Manitoba.

It is hardy to the rest of the prairies, but cannot make it over dry, prairie soil, and needs trees for support. The plant has inconspicuous yellow-green flowers, that when both sexes are present, will produce fruit.

These grape-like berries are considered poisonous, and possibly fatal, to children. The berry has very sharp-ridged pits that can also be irritating or damaging to intestinal tissue.

The Cherokee used the root for skin diseases, as a diuretic and laxative. It was prepared and taken by "weakly females", before or after childbirth, and for a weak stomach and bowels. It was called appropriately Moonroot, or **UDO SA NO E HI**.

The Delaware made a salve for use on chronic sores.

The Omaha Ponca call it Thunder Grapes, or **INGTHAHE-HAZI-I-TA**.

Another name among the Ponca was Grapes of the Ghost. The Pawnee went for the more obvious, less poetic Sore Mouth, or **HAKAKUT**.

At one time, it was used as a substitute for sarsaparilla in "root" beers.

The Blister Beetle, *Chauliognathus marginatus,* aggressively attacks and shreds *Potentilla* and other flowers for pollen and nectar. When it lands on the small flowers of Moonseed it carefully takes the pollen, and flicks the grains from the anther. It then licks nectar from the base of female flowers without injuring the ovary. Clever.

MEDICINAL

CONSTITUENTS- Alkaloids make up 2.2% of the plant by dry weight, and include acutimine, acutimidine, (-)viburnitol, daurinoline, dauricine, magnoflorine, dehydrocheilanthifoline, N'-demethyldauricine, N'-methyl-lindcarpine; vinetine (oxyacanthine) and berberine.

Millspaugh noted that the use of Moonseed by early practitioners was very similar to sarsaparilla. It was an official drug in the *US Pharmacopoeia* from 1882 to 1905 as a tonic and diuretic.

Earlier, various Native healers used the root for scrofula, or tuberculosis of the neck lymph glands; while early settlers used it as a diuretic for strangury in their horses.

Dr. King noted "indications seem to point to its probable value in leucocythaemia, especially when the spleen is prominently involved."

Dr. Brown, in 1875 wrote, "yellow parilla seems to possess one virtue which is paramount to all others, it is essentially and particular anti-syphilitic, anti-scrofulous, anti-mercurial".

Dr. Cook voiced similar opinion, stating "in small doses, its action is chiefly manifested upon the respiratory passages, where it increases expectoration and gives a feeling of stimulation to the lungs...the stomach is fairly improved by it, and the hepatic apparatus and smaller bowels distinctly influenced, whence it will lead to free discharge of bile and to fair evacuations of the bowels.

Its general glandular action makes it valuable in scrofula, secondary syphilis, mercurial rheumatism, indolent ulcers and similar low conditions...Most commonly it is combined with more relaxing articles such as *Rumex, Fraxinus, Celastrus* and *Arctium lappa."*

Alma Hutchens, in her somewhat erratic book, notes that it is useful "for all diseases arising from inheritary (sic) or acquired impurities of the system. It exerts its influence principally on the gastric and salivary glands and is found expressly beneficial in cases of adhesive inflammation and where it is found necessary to break up organized deposits and hasten disintegration of unwanted tissue."

Bolyard, in his book, *Medicinal Plants and Home Remedies of Appalachia* gives the following recipe.

"One span of (Moonseed root) is boiled in a quart of water until one half pint of liquid remains. One half pint of whisky and a heaping tablespoon of sulfur is added to this. One spoonful is taken before each meal until it is all used."

Grieve, in A Modern Herbal, noted Moonseed contained berberine.

She writes “in small doses it is a tonic, diuretic, laxative and alterative. In larger doses, it increases the appetite and action of the bowels; in full doses, it purges and causes vomiting.

Externally, the decoction has been applied as an embrocation in cutaneous and gouty affections... in powder is recommended as a nervine and is considered superior to Sarsaparilla taken in does of 1-3 grains, three times daily.”

It is a superior laxative bitter, considered very useful for scrofula, cutaneous, rheumatic, syphilitic, mercurial, and arthritic diseases; also for dyspepsia, chronic inflammation of the viscera and in general debility.

She forgot to note that light increases in heart pulse will be noticed in large doses as well.

Dauricine is used as an anti-arrhythmic agent in China. It has been shown to inhibit platelet aggregation in work by Tong et al, *Yao Xue Xue Bao* 1989 24:2.

More recent work confirms dauricine’s effect in cardiac arrhythmia. Qian, *Acta Pharmacol Sin* 2002 23:12.

The herb has influence on the spleen and may be of use in some forms of leukocytosis.

Dauricine is an isoquinoline alkaloid with anesthetic, anti-inflammatory and weak curare-like activity. It is anti-arrhythmic and cardio-protective.

It is a platelet activating factor (PAF) receptor ligand. Viburnitol is also present in yarrow.

The alkaloid acutamine has been shown to inhibit growth of human T cells.

Oxyacanthine, also found in *Mahonia, Magnolia* and *Ranunculus* species, is anti-microbial to *Bacillus subtilis* and *Colpidium colpuda*, as well as, an adrenalin antagonist and vasodilator.

It is one of the few bitter tonics that does not contain tannic or gallic acid.

HOMEOPATHY

Moonseed (*M. canadense*) is a remedy for migraine, and is associated with restlessness and dreams. There may be spinal pain, with a dryness and itchiness all over, and dryness of the mouth and throat.

The head has pressure from within outward, with stretching and yawning, and pains down the back. There may be sick headaches, with pain in the forehead and temples, moving toward the occiput. The tongue is swollen, with copious saliva.

The legs are sore, as is bruised, with pain in the thighs, elbows and shoulders.

They feel so weak, empty and hollow that is as if the whisper of death is heard.

Low spirited, but attend to business with rapidity. Quick tempered, irritable, surly, ill-natured and stubborn.

DOSE- Third potency. Taylor did self-experiment with tincture in 1867, and Graham with 1x trituration of menispermine in same year.

SEED OIL

The fruit seeds contain 16% oil composed mainly of octadecadienoic acid (46%), oleic acid, 29%, and octadecatrienoic acid (25%).

PERSONALITY TRAITS

A fundamental theme of Menispermaceae is oversensitivity. Plants in general are sensitive to outside influences. Some plant families, like Menispermaceae, are more sensitive than most.

Menispermaceae are sensitive to numerous things such as emotions, pain, noise and touch..[and]...especially sensitive to the suffering of others and those who need care.

Generally, Menispermaceae have a strong sense of self-reliance and responsibility. They think everyone has the duty to take care of themselves, yet when confronted with the unfortunate, they can't help but to take on that responsibility too. Though weighed down by the duty, they would feel guilty if they didn't.

Taking on the responsibility of care and tending to those in need lead to emotional over-reactions. They are too caring, too concerned and too sensitive to the situation of seeing someone ill. They can't moderate or modulate their impressions and reactions. They have to react, to care, to move, to overdo, overextend and overwork.

The strain causes either outbursts of irritability or a complete collapse to the extent that they are now as ill and debilitated as they initially were driven to help. Only reducing the underlying sensitivity will allow them to moderate their reactions and offer the kind of assistance that is truly beneficial to all concerned, especially themselves.

VERMEULEN

MYTHS AND LEGENDS

Long ago it rained for many days and the land was flooded for miles around. The Indians has to go about in canoes and food was becoming scarce. They appealed to the Chief to know what to do.

The chief said, "Make ropes of the Moonseed vine half as long as a boy can walk in one sun. Put the ropes in your canoes and get into them. Wait until the water gets as high as yon rocky height, then attach one end of the rope to the rock and the other end to the canoes".

The Indians fell to work twisting the fibers of the vine, but they grew tired and stopped when the ropes were still short. All but Goplobet who worked on and on, until he had obeyed the chief's instructions.

He wound his rope up and it filled the canoe. The Indians waited until the water had risen to its highest, then tied their canoes to the rock. As the waters went down, one short rope snapped, then another, until all the canoes but Goplobet's, were adrift.

Soon the canoes were scattered all over the earth and that is why there are so many tribes of Indians. But Goplobet stayed in the same country and became a great chief and had many children. **GUILLET**

RECIPES

TINCTURE- 10-40 drops as needed. For a bitter tonic take 5-10 in water before meals. The dry root tincture is made at 1:5 with 70% alcohol.

DECOCTION- 1-4 ounces three times daily.

DR. CHRISTOPHER'S ALTERATIVE COMPOUND- Take two parts each of red clover, moonseed and burdock root, and combine it with one part mullein. Simmer in water, until reduced by half. Dosage is four ounces three to four times daily.

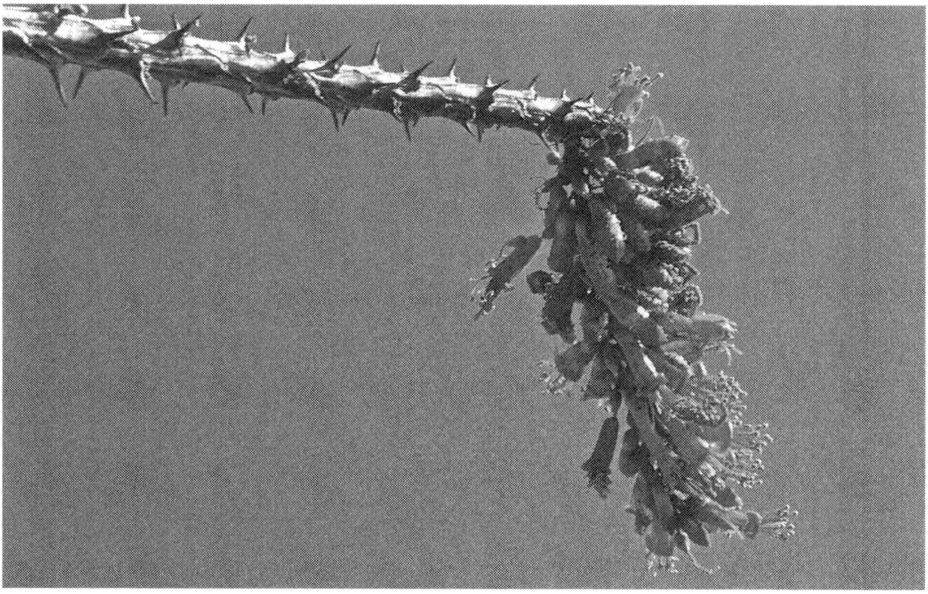

Ocotillo flower and stem

OCOTILLO
JACOB'S STAFF
COACH WHIP

(*Fouquieria splendens* Engelm.)

PARTS USED- limbs, flowers

Ocotillo is from the Mexican Spanish **OCOTE** meaning, little pine, in turn from the Nahuatl **OCOTL**, a torch made from pine. Fouquieria is named in honor of Pierre Fouquier, a 19th century French physician. Splendens means shiny, glossy or beautiful and has same root as splendid, splendour and splendant.

It is a bizarre looking plant of the southwestern desert. It is long-lived perennial that can survive its hot, dry environment for sixty to seventy years. A large specimen can have up to one hundred spiny stems that rise straight up from the root.

When the spring rains come to the desert, the small waxy oval leaves poke out. In fact, any time of sufficient rain, will trigger a burst of leaves that quickly die and fade in the scorching sun. The leaves turn into spines that cover the stem top to bottom.

It is common to the Sonoran, Mojave and Chichuahuan deserts.

The dried stems make interesting walking sticks, fence posts, etc. The resin and wax are gathered to condition leather.

Traditionally, the Hispanic New Mexicans have used ocotillo for sore throat, tonsillitis and to stimulate stalled menstruation. The Cahuilla decocted the root to treat irritating, moist coughs in the elderly. It is a mild expectorant that helps move thick mucus up and out. It also sedates dry, spasmodic coughs, combining well with scarlet mallow.

The Apache used either fresh or dried flowers for sore, inflamed muscles. The seeds and flowers were added to various meals for color and flavour.

MEDICINAL

CONSTITUENTS- bark- adoxoside, fouquierol, iso-fouquierol, ocotillol, adoxosidic acid
Leaf- 6-beta-hydroxy splendoside, 7-beta-hydroxy splendoside, galioside, isoquercitin, rutin, splendoside
Leaf and bark- asperocotillin, asperuloside, caffeic acid, kaempferol, leucocyandin, p-coumarin, ellagic acid, cinnamic acid, quercitin, scopoletin
Root-dammarendiol

Ocotillo is first, and foremost, a pelvic lymphatic decongestant. That is, it helps move congestion of the lymphatic and venous system associated with hemorrhoids, prostatitis, benign prostatic hyperplasia, and mesenteric stagnation. Cervical varicosities and heavily congested, edemic conditions of lower trunk are relieved.

It is suggested that the stagnant, cottage cheese-like congestion is thinned and portal vein circulation to the liver is restored.

Michael Moore said it better than anyone. Ocotillo "is useful for those symptoms that arise from pelvic fluid congestion, both lymphatic and venous. It is absorbed from the intestines into the mesenteric lymph system by way of the lacteals of the small intestinal lining; this stimulates better visceral lymph drainage into the thoracic duct and improves dietary fat absorption into the lymph system.

With fewer dietary lipids going into the liver by the portal blood, there is less tendency for the intestinal blood to back up (portal hypertension) and less stagnation in the pelvis and upper thighs. Most hemorrhoids are helped by Ocotillo, as are cervical varicosities and benign prostate enlargements.

The same is true of a frequent need to urinate, with dull ache but no inflammation of the urethra, and the kinds of varicose veins and piles worsened by constipation or poor digestion." It combines well with figwort and cleavers.

FLOWER ESSENCES

Ocotillo flower essence is for disembodied spiritual experiences not fully owned by the conscious soul.

It is for excessive psychic "fire" leading to emotional reactivity, psychic projection and distortion, or various forms of anger and violence, alcoholism and other drug addictions. In the positive state, Ocotillo forces are grounded and integrated in the core individuality of the soul. **FLOWER ESSENCE SOCIETY**

Ocotillo is for individuals who have subconscious or unexpressed feelings that erupt in uncontrolled ways. Ocotillo gives insight into and acceptance of our emotions without feeling victimized by them. There is trust in the knowledge that we are unconditionally loved, protected and guided. **DESERT ALCHEMY**

RECIPES

FRESH BARK TINCTURE- 30-60 drops three times daily in ice cold water. Make from the fresh bark at 1:4 ratio with 70-80% alcohol.

BARK DECOCTION- 4-6 ounces up to three times daily ice cold.

PIPSISSEWA
PRINCE'S PINE
(*Chimaphila umbellata* [L.] Nutt.)
(*C. umbellata* [L.] W. Barton)
(*Pyrola corymbosa* [Pursh) Bertol.)
(*Pyrola umbellata* L.)
PARTS USED- root, leaves, flowers

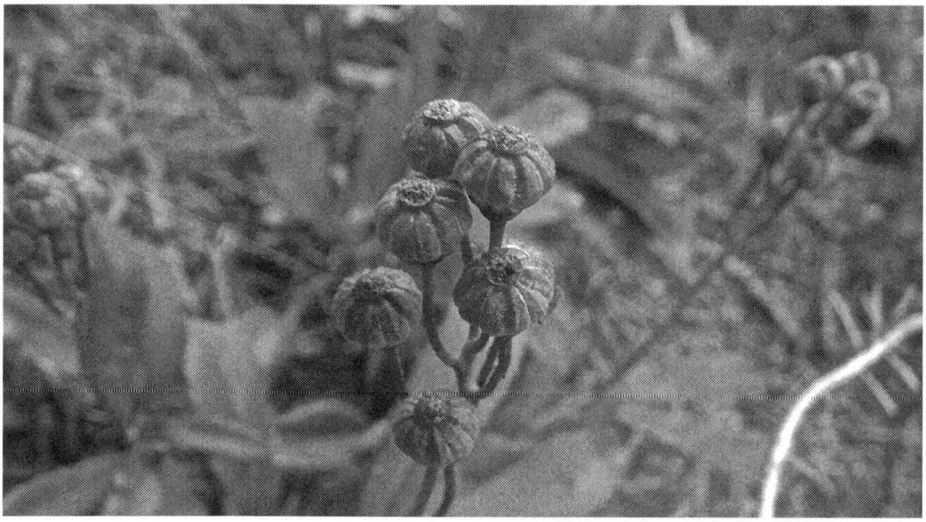

Seed pods of Prince's Pine

Pipsissewa is from the Cree **PIPISISKWEU** meaning, "it breaks it into small pieces", and refers to the leaves containing a substance that breaks down kidney stones.

It is one of my favourite examples of herbal onomatopoeia, which refers to the word describing the act of urination. The Abenaki name is **KPI PSKW AHSAWE** means flower of the woods.

Chimaphila is derived from the Greek **CHEIMA** meaning winter, and **PHILOS** meaning, love, in reference to the evergreen leaves. Umbellata describes the flower cluster or umbel.

Pipsissewa is common throughout the pine forests of the Rockies and in the Cypress Hills of southern Alberta. Native people of the province used the plant for a variety of problems involving inflammation of the skin, kidneys and menstrual cycle.

The Cree of northern Saskatchewan call it **AMISKWATHOWIPAK**, meaning beaver tail leaf. Decoctions of the whole plant were used for stabbing pains in the chest (angina pectoris), backache, coughing up of blood, and various fever and pain states.

The Blackfeet dried the leaves of **O-MAKSI-KA-KA-SIN**, and used them as part of smoking mixtures; while the Chippewa decocted the root and used the water to soothe sore eyes; or part of a combination to treat gonorrhea.

The Anishinaabemowin names are **GAAGIGEBAG** meaning everlasting leaf, and **MAKOONSOMIN** for pipsissewa berry.

The Catawba called it Fire Flower, and used it for backaches.

The Karuk name **XUNYEEPSHURUK HITIHAN** means, "one who is under tan oak trees", which is true in that part of the world. The leaves and stems were steeped into a tea for bladder complaints.

Sam Hill, Onondaga herbalist from the Six Nations Reserve, had this to say about the herb in 1912.

"When a pregnant women feels feverish and drowsy, she is not sick, her baby is. Make a small bundle of pipsissewa about one inch thick using the whole plant. Put this in one half quart of water to steep. Take a cupful four times a day until it is used up."

The Wasco of Oregon decocted whole plant to treat tuberculosis.

It was used with wild sarsaparilla as part of traditional recipes for root beer.

The raw leaves can even be eaten, although somewhat stringy and fibrous. In parts of Appalachia, the leaves are chewed to relieve heartburn.

The fresh leaves were bruised and applied to rheumatic pains, and scrofula. A reddening and blistering of the skin can result, however, from prolonged application.

The leaf and root decoctions are red brown with a clean bitter taste that changes to sort of sweet taste, with no sign of wintergreen flavour.

Samuel Thomson used it as a tonic for kidneys and urinary tract, while Dr. Cook used it for vaginal and uterine weakness.

Felter used it for elder people with "chronic cystitis with a pinkish or reddish sediment of mucus, pus, blood and brick dust in the urine", and prostatitis.

Dr. Eli Jones suggested its use for breast cancer in large breasted women, where the lymphatic glands are involved. Other Eclectic physicians used it as part of formulas for prostate and bladder cancer.

Various tribes ate the berries as stomachics, or digestive tonics.

Pipsissewa extracts are used as "secret" flavour components today for root beer and sarsaparilla soft drinks, as well as candy, frozen dairy, baked goods (290 ppm), gelatins, puddings and sweet sauces (365 ppm). It is wild-crafted extensively, and rapidly disappearing from the Pacific Northwest.

Pipsissewa was carried traditionally to attract money. When crushed and combined with rosehips and violet flowers, and burned, it was said to draw good spirits for magical aid.

The herb is used in traditional Chinese Medicine, as a diuretic, anti-fungal and to relieve stomach, tooth and after birth pains. It is called **MEI LI CAO**.

The closely related *P. maculata* is European, but nearly identical in composition. It is commonly found throughout the Appalachians.

In Germany it was called **HARNKRAUT**, meaning Urine Weed; alluding to the plant's urinary activity.

Paracelsus wrote of the plant "for wounds, for old weeping injuries...to stop abdominal fluxes...and for fresh wounds, there is hardly a remedy in greater repute for healing these."

MEDICINAL

CONSTITUENTS- flavonoids including hyperoside, quercitin, and avicularin; arbutin (7.5%), isohomo-arbutin, homoarbutin, hyperin, avicularin, kaempferol, chinic acid, urson, ericolin; taraxasterin, sitosterin, renifolin, hentriacontane, nonacosane ($C_{29}H_{60}$), ursolic acid, toluquinol, silicic acid, sufphuric acid, epicatechin gallate, methyl salicylate, kaempferol, quercitin, naphthoquinones such as chimphilin (2%); tannins, including epicatechol gallate (4%), beta amyrin, pectin, gums and bitters.

Pipsissewa is a valuable cool and dry herb for scanty urine and urinary infections. It is somewhat less astringent than bearberry, but a stronger diuretic with less stomach irritation due to less tannin. It does, however, remove gravel and uric acid, and relieves chronic prostate irritation in the manner of bearberry.

It was considered at one time to be a specific for men over fifty, suffering from chronic bladder irritation.

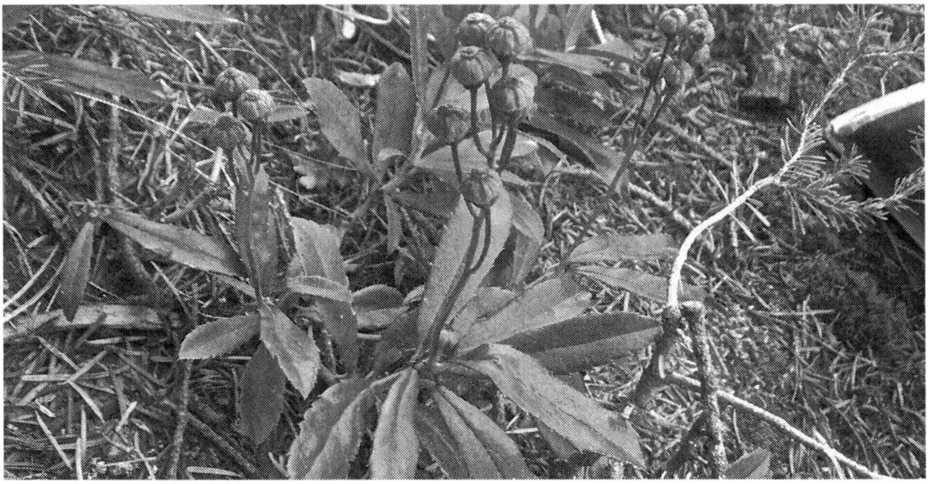

Pipsissewa plants in seed - Note the evergreen leaves

Various Eclectic physicians, including Felter, Ellingwood and Lloyd prescribed pipsissewa for burning urination associated with chronic cystitis and prostate congestion.

For chronic nephritis, combine pipsissewa with goldenrod; while lymphatic congestion of the breast calls for the addition of cleavers and red root.

It may be used over the long term for benign prostatic hyperplasia, or enlargement of the prostate, general kidney weakness and mild nephritis. It is used for chronic low-grade infections of bacterial vaginosis and chlamydia, with enlarged lymph glands in the groin.

It may be used concurrently with antibiotics to treat gonorrhea.

Many of the bactericide constituents are excreted as disinfectant substances, making it a valuable plant for chronically suppressed skin eruptions. For swollen and congested lymphatic glands, ovarian cysts, and lipomas (congested fat lumps under the skin), it can be used internally as a cool decoction and externally as a poultice or wash for ulcerous sores, tumours, blisters and swelling. Inflammation of the cervical lymph plexus is relieved.

Michael Moore suggested "it is an effective alterative for lingering skin conditions characterized by dry, flaky inflammation, vague aching in the joints, and frequent urination at night."

Matthew Wood added. “Pipsissewa is a great “eliminator of kapha”, if I may coin a phrase. It warms and activates the lymphatics and kidneys, the carriers and dispersers of water in the body…It is indicated in the sluggishness, water retention, and weight gain of middle age. It is indicated when the tongue is swollen and coated white in the middle. This might be an indication of ‘spleen yang deficiency’ in traditional Chinese medicine, a category similar to ‘scrofula’ in old-time Western medicine.”

Ursolic acid inhibits COX-2, thereby alleviating pain and inflammation. Dr. Hale, an Eclectic physician wrote. “It is chiefly in chronic rheumatism that its curative powers have been most observed”.

Laboratory studies have confirmed pipsissewa’s benefit in hypoglycemia, and its tonic effect in late-onset diabetes. Arbutin is not only anti-bacterial and anti-tussive, but inhibits insulin degradation.

It relieves rheumatoid aliments, and restores mobility in rundown and debilitated individuals.

As a hot infusion, it helps reduce fevers due to infection, especially if caught early. Cystitis, including interstitial, urethritis, prostatitis, and nephritis all respond better to infusions at body temperature.

Tannic astringency in the herb is of benefit in diarrhea, and internal bleeding such as stomach ulcers, birthing and peridontal disease. Long decoctions create more astringency.

Due to methyl salicylate content and its pain relieving property, the plant is useful for urinary tract infections associated with pain, and postpartum hemorrhage.

Chimaphilin stimulates phagocytes, one of our non-specific immune cells, at low doses. Harbourne et al, 1993.

It was first isolated in 1860 by Samuel Fairbanks, upon distillation. Its structure is similar to vitamin K, and several studies confirm reduction of clotting time.

Chimaphilin shows greatest activity against *Staphylococcus aureus*, moderate benefit against *E. coli* and *Candida albicans*, and some activity against *Shigella sonnei*, Ambrogi et al, *British J Pharmacy* 1970 40.

Anti-fungal activity was noted by Steffen and Peschel, *Planta Medica* 1975 27.

Work by Towers et al, at the U of British Columbia found aerial parts active against all nine fungal species tested. Ethanol extracts of the whole plant show activity against *Candida albicans*. Jones et al, *J Ethnopharm* 2000 73.

Chimaphilin is a powerful anti-fungal with significant activity against organisms responsible for dandruff. Galván et al, *Phytochem* 2007 Oct 23.

Chimaphilin, *in vitro*, inhibits platelet aggregation induced by collagen and ADP, and is active on atrial tissue from guinea pigs.

Bishop & MacDonald *Can J Botany* 1951 29, tested 209 plant species, and found *C. umbellata* ether extracts one of the most effective against *S. aureus* of all plants they tested. Only Sweet Gale (*Myrica gale*) in alcohol showed more inhibition.

Some Eastern Native healers combine it with mint as a tea for stomach cancer.

Work by Oka et al, *Phytomed* June 20 2007 found a combination of Pipsissewa, Aspen Poplar, *Pulsatilla pratensis*, Horsetail and wheat germ oil reduced benign prostatic hypertrophy. The individual constituents did not show any effect, and yet the combination showed significant improvement.

The proprietary compound Eviprostat® is used in Japan and Europe for treatment of BPH, or benign prostatic hyperplasia.

The fresh leaves are good counter-irritant, if poulticed and left for at least 30 minutes. Use for arthritis, rheumatism and associated congestions, but caution against blistering of skin is advised.

Some herbals suggest you can substitute *Uva ursi* for this herb. In terms of astringency, this is true, but it lacks the analgesic effect of methyl salicylate. In this case use two parts bearberry and one part birch twigs as a substitute.

Like Uva ursi, the content of arbutin is from 17-22%. Arbutin, of course, converts to hydroquinone after metabolic or bacterial conversion, and is anti-bacterial.

The flavonoids and their glycosides show anti-inflammatory activity, as does beta sitosterol. The latter, however, is insoluble in water and minimally soluble in alcohol.

The whole plant suppressed oxidative stress in rats with surgically induced bladder outlet obstruction. Oka et al, *The Journal of Urology* 2009 182 382-90.

Watkins, in the *Eclectic Med Journal* 1902 62 found the fluid extract more active after sitting for 6-12 months. With time, the liquid becomes more gelatinized, with patients reporting better results from the aged product. Not sure why.

HOMEOPATHY

Pipsissewa acts principally on the uro-genital tract, and lymphatic glands. For bladder infections with notable mucous in both acute and chronic conditions, it is very useful. There may be scanty urine, with lots of ropy, mucous sediment. The prostate may be inflamed, leading to scanty and burning urine, with high sugar content possible.

The female labia may be inflamed and swollen, with or without vaginal pain. The breast may have painful tumours, with unexplained milk secretion; and more common in women with large, cystic, painful breasts.

In males, there may be prostatic enlargement with loss of seminal fluid.

Incipient and progressive eye cataracts may be arrested in their growth.

Blue rings around eyes, pain around teeth and jaw. Tongue sore and full of little vesicles.

The symptoms are worse on the left side of the body, in damp weather, and from sitting on cold.

DOSE- Tincture to third potency. Mother tincture is prepared from the whole fresh plant in flower. Provings by Jeanes in 1840 and Bute in 1856. Clinical observations by Hering and Stauffer.

FLOWER ESSENCE

Pipsissewa is the flower essence for clearing ambivalence. It is a decision maker, helping us choose as a responsible act. It also helps resolve the frustration around having made a choice which seems not to turn out the way we thought it would. Instead of wasting energy bewailing where we find ourselves, the essence will help move us to the point of power in the present where we can make a new choice.

Physically, it impacts upon the brain and awakens that area involved in choice. It affects the throat and solar plexus chakras. **PACIFIC**

SPIRITUAL PROPERTIES

Pipsissewa is a powerful healer for deep release. It creates a spiral of energy in the abdomen that is ongoing. Blockages of spiritual growth such as fear and guilt are released. The cleansing is from the heart down, and negative thought forms are released. It does not, however, have the energetics to release past life patterns.

If in an intimate relationship, both of you may take pipsissewa to release negative energy and help develop greater love. There may be initial irritation, but then an emotional cleansing takes place.

The whorl pattern of the leaves is representative of spiral energy. The etheric body is cleansed and a few hours after taking the tea, the etheric is strengthened.

Mars, and its negative effect when in opposition or squared are eased.

GURUDAS

Pipsissewa's key word is awareness; both self-awareness and environmental awareness. It enhances the awareness of every piece of information, of every stimulus, in every sense. **MULDERS**

PERSONALITY TRAITS

As a child, the pipsissewa type suffers from chronic lymphatic congestion. The tonsils and/or appendix have been removed, or as a teenager, mononucleosis has affected the spleen.

Later in life there is poor skin with lymphatic congestion and sluggishness. The kidneys are weak, and there may be prostate inflammation in the male.

On the negative side, the pipsissewa person is prone to fears and lack of self-esteem. They may rely on others for approval, and choose careers or marriage partners that reflect that internal imbalance.

On the positive side, the pipsissewa person learns at an early age to care for themselves. They may be overly sensitive as children, and as adults learn to not take things personally.

They also recognize the symptoms of congestion that lead to stagnation on a physical and emotional plane. **PRAIRIE DEVA**

BOTANICA POETICA

Pipsissewa, an Evergreen
Helps to keep the urine clean
With its tannins, it's astringent
Salicylates and quinones in it
For urinary disinfection
Also calms the inflammation
And if the prostate's oversized
Give Pipsissewa a try
A bitter tonic, diuretic
Use the leaf for joints arthritic
Chimaphila Umbellata
Cleanse the blood and the liver
Take this herb for UTI
Also known as Prince's Pine
It's endangered so make haste
Don't overuse and create waste
Truth be known to all who care
Though it smells rather fair
The infusion as my tea
Did not taste so good to me!
SYLVIA CHATROUX MD

RECIPES

DECOCTION- Take one heaping tablespoon of dried leaf to one pint of hot water. Simmer twenty minutes. Drink at body temperature for skin or urogenital infections, cold for lymphatic, lipomas and breast affections, and hot for fever conditions. Four to eight ounces 3 times daily. The fresh leaf tea is irritating to the kidneys.

POWDER- 30-90 grains daily

TINCTURE- fresh preferred- 15-60 drops in divided doses daily in water. For a dry plant tincture use a 1:5 ratio with 50% alcohol. For fresh tincture, my own preference, use a 1:2 ratio of 60%. For bladder cancer use ten drops in large amount of water up to three times a day.

In general, only use for ten days, take a five-day break and repeat. For urinary tract infections, combine with equal parts of uva-ursi and usnea/lomatium- 90 drops 4x daily in warm water with pinch of baking soda.

For kidney stones take two tsps twice daily in cool water. For pulmonary edema, use 10ml of fresh leaf tincture per litre of water. Drink in divided doses.

CAUTION- urine may have a green tone, it is harmless. Do not use during pregnancy or lactation.

FLUID EXTRACT- One tsp three times daily.

A method for determining chimaphilin content can be found in *Pharmazie* 1997 52:2 based on work of Michelitsch.

POKEROOT
(*Phytolacca decandra* [L.] A. Gray)
(*P. americana* L.)
PARTS USED- root, leaf, berries

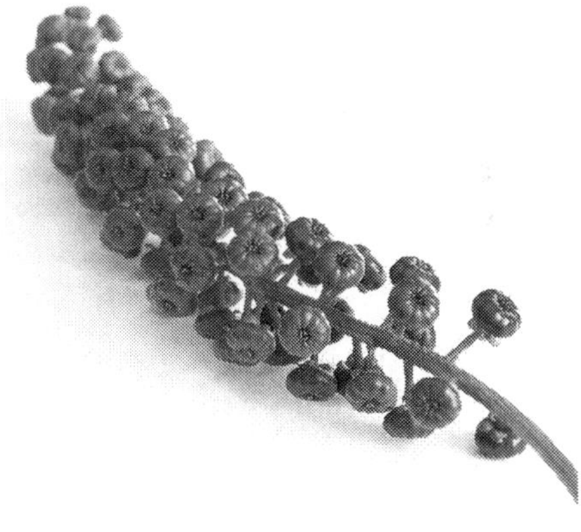
American Pokeweed

Phytolacca is from the Greek for plant (phyto) and French word for lake, as in the color. It is not the sky blue you would assume but a dark red. Or it may be from the Persian-Arabic **LAKK** meaning, lacquer. Decandra is Greek and refers to the ten stamens. Andros means "male" as in androgen.

Poke is from **POCAN**, a plant that yields yellow or red dye. The Algonquian word **PAK** means blood, hence puccoon. Blood root is red puccoon, and goldenseal is yellow puccoon.

The plant has many common names including poke, skoke, scoke, pocan, cokan, chongras, cocum and polk. The latter name led to supporters of James Polk, running for president in 1844, wearing pokeweed leaves as the emblem of support.

Natives made a blue stain for their splint baskets from the berry.

The Cherokee infused berries for arthritis and rheumatism and cold infusions of dry root were taken for kidney problems. The Delaware added the root to mixtures as a stimulant and blood purifier. Further north, the Iroquois decocted the steams for chest colds, and applied poultices to bruises and bunions. It was tied in a poplar tree as a love medicine. The Mahuna used a leaf wash for acne and blackheads, while the Mi'kmaq used the infusion for bleeding wounds.
The Mohegan applied mashed berries to sore breasts, while the Rappahannock cured hemorrhoids using decocted root steam.

It was at one time listed in the *US Pharmacopoeia*.

The leaves have been prized as an edible, but only after two changes of water. The town of Harlan, Kentucky has an annual Poke Sallet Festival. A favorite is fresh leaves sautéed in bacon with black-eyed peas and cornbread. It produces fresh greens all year round where it grows from Ontario to the Maritime provinces, and from Minnesota to the Gulf States. On a recent visit to South Carolina, I was promised a feed of poke but alas my time in that beautiful state ran out before I could have a feed.

The thickened leaf juice was traditionally applied to skin cancer and indolent ulcers. Leaf decoction washes help relieve swollen hemorrhoids. See root oil below for preparation into suppositories and external breast application.

The root can be put into a root cellar and will produce fresh shoots all winter long. The fruit is edible, but the seeds are toxic.

In TCM, the plant is known as **SHANG LU**. The energetics are bitter, cooling and toxic, and used for edema, full distention of gastrointestinal or respiratory system, sore throat and dysuria.

MEDICINAL

CONSTITUENTS- root- various triterpenoid saponins, phytolaccoside A-1, D2 and O, aglycones including phytolaccagenin, jaligonic acid, phytolaccagenic acid, asculentic acid, acinosolic acid methyl ester, lectins; phytolaccine, betanidine, betanine, isobetanine, isoprebetanine and prebetanine (alkaloids); bitter resins, isoamericanin A, PAP (pokeweed antiviral protein), alpha spinasterol, histamine, GABA, phytolaccic acid, formic acid, tannins, potassium formate, calcium oxalate.

The root is slightly pungent, bitter, dry and sweet. It is stimulating, softening, dissolving and neutral in nature, especially in cases of torpor and lack of tissue tone.

It is very useful for swollen lymphatic glands, including hardened nodules that are painful and swollen. This includes breast conditions that are swollen, inflamed and engorged, especially during PMS.

Early Eclectic physicians, including Ellingwood, considered it an "alterative influencing the glands". Individuals with pale mucosa, ulceration and swollen glands were specific.

Peter Holmes puts it well. "Poke root is a systemic *resolvent detoxicant* remedy with particular affinity for the exocrine glandular system, especially the lymphatic circulation.

Blue iris, especially Hydrogenoid, iris constitutions, take note!...The remedy is especially useful for subjects that badly need resolution of chronically enlarged, painful, hard lymph glands, eczema with chronic dryness and irritation, and hardening/depository disorders such as cirrhosis, fibrocystic breasts and lipomas."

Matthew Wood writes. "It has a special affinity for the glandular system. It is relevant when there are stagnant, swollen lymphatics, swollen sore throat, diphtheria, mastitis or breast problems in general. As is common in remedies that affect the lymphatic glands, there is also a powerful influence on endocrine regulation."

It is best combined, in small amounts, with cleavers or an alterative such as burdock root.

Poke root is an excellent anti-inflammatory and useful in lymphadenitis, laryngitis, pericarditis and burns. It is anti-fungal, anti-viral and increases lymphocyte activity.

A lectin and toll-like receptors in pokeweed activate human B lymphocytes. Bekeredjian-Ding I et al, *PLoS One* 2012 7:1.

Cold sores and genital herpes respond to an external wash as do cervical and anal warts when used as a douche or retention enema. An anti-viral protein shows broad activity *in vitro*, against herpes simplex, influenza and poliovirus. The protein shuts down ribosomal ATP in cells affected by HIV. Aron GM & JD Irvin, *Antimicrob Agents Chemother* 1980 17:6 1032-3.

Inflamed "itis" conditions are relieved including tonsillitis, mastitis, laryngitis, sinusitis, conjunctivitis, otitis, stomatitis, parotitis, orchitis, ovaritis and osteomyelitis. The latter is of particular note, as musculo-skeletal conditions including cancerous diseases of the bones and spine may be helped. The herb possesses anti-histamine action and GABA that may reduce hypertension. The tonsils have red spots, the throats is blue or red, with a pain upon swallowing that travels to ears. Eustachian tube inflammation with tonsillitis call for poke root.

Breast conditions, including acute mastitis, benign lumps and cancers all respond to internal and external application.

Extracts changed gene expression in colon cancer cell lines. Maness L et al, *Phytotherapy Research* 2014 28:2 219-23.

In the 18th century, Dr. Clapp recommended the root to treat syphilis, commonly called clap. Hmmm. Talk about bringing your work home.

The root is also useful in various rheumatic conditions associated with damp cold including synovial and ligament inflammations, arthritis, gout and neuralgia. Combine black cohosh and poke root with a bit of prickly ash for fibromyalgia.

Combine with ocotillo for pelvic congestion and swollen glands in groin. Or combine with lemon balm for deep-seated coughs with mucus.

Dr. Jones combined thuja, wild indigo and pokeroot in his Cancer drops. William Mitchell suggested two parts Iris, one part Phytolacca, one part Lobelia and two parts dandelion root and leaf for lymphatic stasis. Thirty drops in large glass of water three times daily. He also liked three parts Echinacea, three parts Astragalus root and one part poke root for immune enhancement, at 60 drops three times daily.

In his book, *Plant Medicine in Practice*, he mentions Dr. Bastyr using poke root to treat lymphogranuloma venereum. Dosage was 10 drops four times daily. He also used the herb for fibrosing proctitis with 2000 IU of vitamin E daily.

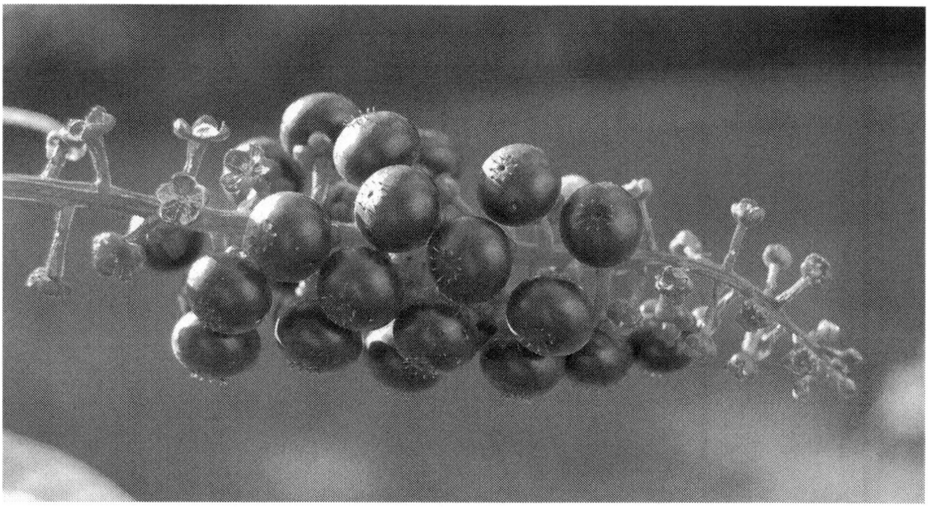

Pokeweed berries

HOMEOPATHY

POKE ROOT

There is a sense of indifference and aversion to work. The patient may speak in silly voices or exhibit childish behavior. They can be rude. Symptoms are worse at night, from damp or cold weather, and pains appear suddenly and can be like an electric shock, radiating all over body.

Tendons behind knee feel shortened. Erythema and itching of skin from exposure to sun, especially after winter.

Nipples may be sore, fissured or pain from nipple all over body when nursing. Breast is hard, nodular and lumpy. Cancer of breast. Ovarian neuralgia on right side.

Kent considered this a syphilitic remedy. Hering found "complete shamelessness and indifference to exposure of her person".

At one time was used for the buboes of *Yersinia pestis*.

DOSE- Tincture to third potency. Externally for mastitis. Provings by Hering on 9 males with tincture, 1X, 2X, 3X, 4X, and 10X in 1836; self experimentation by Burt with tincture in 1860s; Fellows with tincture and 1X in 1864; Marshall with tincture in 1869; Cooley with powdered root in same year; Bannan with four provers with 30C in 1999 and clinical observations by Hering, Mangialavori and Dorothy Shepherd.

A recent study found mother tincture and 30C, 200C, 1M and 10M dilutions show activity against MCF-7 human breast carcinoma.

Both mother tinctures and homeopathic preparation produced cytotoxicity and decease in cell proliferation. Arora S et al, *Homeopathy* 2013 102(4):274-82.

Poke berry is for sore throats and treating obesity.

DOSE- as above.

ROOT OIL

Use a 1:7 ratio of fresh green root to good carrier oil. Put in crock pot, lid off, at lowest heat for six or more hours. Strain. Use poke root oil on affected skin conditions as well as swollen glands, indolent ulcers and cancerous breasts that show purple coloration. Use gloves when handling green roots.

FLOWER ESSENCES

Pokeweed essence is for people who wallow in depths of their emotions. Especially for sad, depressed and mournful individuals. It balances base chakra releasing emotions and spirituality stored therein. Strong opening and enhancing effect of kundalini affecting seven chakras along the spine and relevant etheric fluidium. It also binds nadis to the meridians. **PEGASUS**

PERSONALITY TRAITS

Poke root is especially suited to large, bulky persons, with large glands, large breasts, who are poky—they are continually exhausted and want to fling themselves down in a chair or bed. They come home, throw their tools or clothes on the floor, and lie apathetically; meanwhile their surroundings become a pigsty.

Such behavior is not uncommon in teenagers, going through hormonal and glandular development, and phytolacca is an excellent remedy for "lazy teenagers"—or for "lazy teenagers of any age." Poke root is indicated in fevers where glands are involved and apathy and exhaustion take over, and in conditions where the glandular stasis is so great that the blood and nerves are blocked, resulting in lymphatic swelling, purple and red coloration, and acute nerve pain. **WOOD**

How much more negative could the 'Phytolacca' person become, you may well ask! Aching, lumpy and with skin breaking out at odd times, surely there is suffering enough. The most negative aspect of a chronic 'Phytolacca' is that symptoms may be so deeply reinforced and part of the birthright that they *resist* all manner of medical treatment, and may also be very slow, grudgingly loosening little by little, under naturopathic treatments as well. There are no quick cures for this person...In desperation, they may take massive amounts of analgesics, anti-inflammatory drugs, and suppressive or replacement hormones (Cortisone preparations) for the rest of their lives.

Positive 'Phytolacca' is aware that at times of extreme peaks and changes in hormonal activity, it is necessary to rest more, to free the mind from extra stresses and concerns, and to adjust gradually to the differences in lifestyle such periods will inevitably produce.

Most important of all, positive 'Phytolacca' adjusts to the inevitability of change—even welcoming changes as proof that life never stands still, and that nothing lasts forever—not even any negative influence of ancestors!

Too often I have heard from rheumatoid patients. 'Well, it's in the family, you know so I must expect it'. There *are* ways to gradually loosen such influences, if they are first recognized.

DOROTHY HALL

Conversely, Karl-Josef Müller has case-based evidence to suggest that Phytolacca befits overly adapted, over-considerate females, whose will to assert themselves has been broken. He says they are females who had a hard, even vicious mother and have replaced her with an overbearing husband. They have adopted an attitude of keeping their mouths shut, of biting their teeth together, of disregarding their own interests.

Müller perceives Phytolacca as a 'vegetable Lac caninum', particularly because of the predilection of both remedies for the female breast, with a variety of illnesses ranging from acute mastitis to PMS accompanied by hard lumps in the breasts to breast cancer. In addition, Müller has observed a love for dogs and a fear of snakes in Phytolacca patients.

VERMEULEN

MATERIA POETICA

Phytolacca, I recall
You helped when I was sore
'Twas at my breast, a nursing child
And I could take no more.
The breast was hard
The nipples cracked
The glands enlarged
With stiffened back
A fever came to me
I wanted warmth, the weather dry
And something cold to drink
I clenched my teeth
And would not eat
'Til you relieved this all
Someone said that I was shameless too
That part, I don't recall!

SYLVIA CHATROUX MD

RECIPES

TINCTURE- dry root 1:5 at 25%. Dosage is 7-10 drops three times daily.

DECOCTION- one to two grams daily in 1:32 ratio. Drink two ounces up to three times daily ice cold.

CAUTION- Do not use during pregnancy, due to possible teratogenic effect. The fresh root can cause skin irritation and blood changes, so wear gloves during harvest.

Do not take for more than two weeks without a break. Do not take while breastfeeding.

Avoid use with immunosuppressive drugs due to its mitogenic effects.

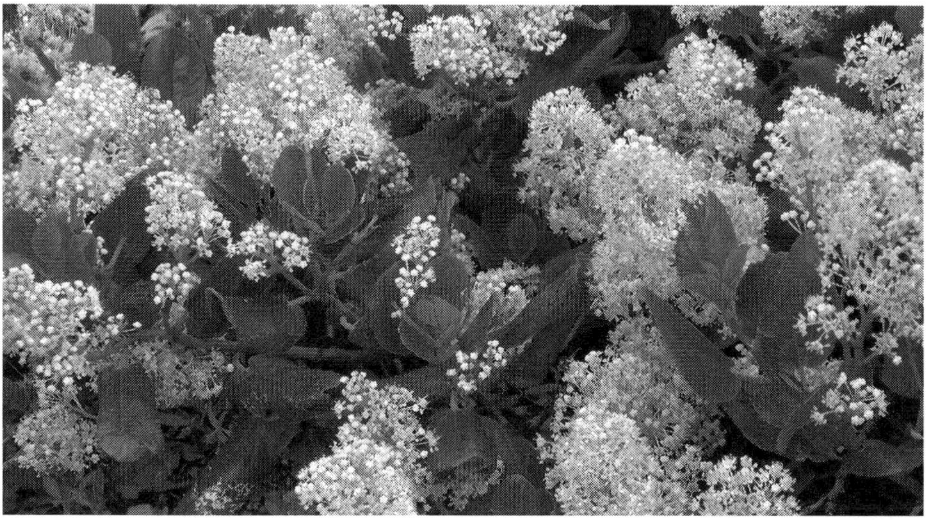

Ceanothus fendleri (Courtesy of Rosalee de la Forêt)

RED ROOT
DEER BRUSH
ELK WEED
SNOWBRUSH
VELVETY BUCKBRUSH
MOUNTAIN BALM
VARNISH BUSH
STICKY LAUREL
(*Ceanothus velutinus* Doug. ex Hook**)**
FENDLER'S BUCKBRUSH
(*C. fendleri* A. Gray**)**
RED STEMMED BUCKBRUSH
RED STEM CEANOTHUS
OREGON TEA TREE
(*C. sanguineus* Pursh.**)**
PARTS USED- root, leaves, flowers

Ceanothus is derived from the Greek via Dioscorides, for an unrelated spiny plant, **KEANOTHOS**.

All species look similar, and range from a tall bush to a sprawling shrub. They share in common a unique, tiny triangular seedpod; with little nodules on the roots that suggest lymphatic nodes.

In the Doctrine of Signatures, a cross section of the root shows a pink-red coming through a pale, serous tan-yellow colouring. It looks like blood flowing through a piece of liver.

Ceanothus species are common in southern British Columbia, into Idaho, Montana and the extreme southwest corner of Alberta. The most studied species, New Jersey Tea (*C. americanus*), is an Eastern species.

The young leaves and twigs of Red-stemmed Buckbrush have a fragrance similar to wintergreen.

The flowers are in large clusters of green-white blossoms honey-sweet, and almost nauseating in large amounts. The flowers will foam into lather when crushed in water.

Red-stemmed Buckbrush was poulticed by Sanpoil people to sores and wounds. Make a poultice of the sapwood and apply it with grease or fat to the affected areas.

The Thompson call it **NAKANAKAI'ELP** meaning, "rotten" or "rotten stink plant", due to its strong, nauseating scent.

The Okanogan used the wood for smoking deer meat, if no other woods were available.

The small seeds of *C. fendleri* were ground into pinole like pine seeds, by various Native tribes. They can remain dormant in the ground for over 200 years, until a forest fire activates them to germination.

Fendler's Buckbrush was used by Navaho healers as sedative for nervousness in combination with other plants.

The leaves can be dried and used as a substitute for black tea; or smoked like tobacco.

Various Native tribes chewed the leaves to relieve inflammations and irritations of the throat and mouth. A leaf tea was used for tuberculosis.

Velvety Buckbrush, or Snowbrush leaf was utilized by members of Karuk as a deodorant. It is known as **UYHURURIP**.

The slimy sap on the inner bark is applied to varicose veins on a moist bandage, or applied directly and covered to keep moist.

The Okanagan and Thompson decocted the stems and leaves and used them both internally and externally for dull pains. The latter call it Rustling Sound, or Rustle Swish, due to the rustling sound made while walking through it.

For arthritis, the roots of false hellebore (*Veratrum*) were combined with redroot as a wash for arthritis. Nancy Turner tells of a case of phlebitis being relieved with a root poultice. Another story tells of a woman who dreamed it was good for cancer. "When you dream of a medicine, what's going to cure you, it's really sacred and you have to do just what they say."

The Shoshone in Wyoming make a beverage tea from the leaves. According to Nickerson, it was used for medical diagnosis as "certain results mean certain things...(and)... the patient breathes out a fresh odor." Natives of Nevada used the leaf tea as a diagnostic tool for illness. After taking the tea, the patient would breathe out a fresh odour for the healer to analyze.

For gonorrhea, the plant branches were boiled for 24 hours with those of buffaloberry (*Shepherdia canadensis*). The patient drank three large cups a day for three or more days to cure milder forms of the disease.

The leaves and twigs were decocted for diarrhea, and ironically, for those who have lost a lot of weight and general illness.

The Shuswap decocted the plants for flu, and smudged the plant to rid their bedding of bugs.

Today, the Secwepemc place the branches on hot stoves to fumigate their homes, the smoke acting as both a disinfectant and insect repellant.

Their anti-fungal activity was used for dandruff, diaper rash and baby powder, according to Dr. Nancy Turner.

The Thompson tribe used snowbrush in combination decoctions for mild forms of gonorrhea, while the Choctaw decocted the roots for lung hemorrhage. The Kootenai made a leaf tea for tuberculosis.

The Flathead of Montana mixed the dried, powdered leaves with fat, and applied this to burns and slow healing sores. The dried powder was used as a baby powder.

The Cherokee used *Ceanothus* species root as a skin lotion to treat cancer.

Red root was first "discovered" in 1835 as "professional medicine" by allopathic physicians. It was utilized by surgeons, in Boston and other cities, as an anti-hemorrhagic astringent to stop bleeding during operations. If they had stopped and looked they would have seen the tincture made from tan yellow roots turns a deep, blood red.

Then, during the Civil War, it developed a reputation for "ague cake", the swollen spleen associated with malaria and intermittent fevers.

This affinity to the glands, spleen and lymphatics was largely unappreciated, with Dr. Cook even commenting that it was "not very powerful or reliable".

New Remedies, a book of indigenous herbal remedies written by Dr. Edwin Hale, mentioned *Ceanothus*. Again it was overlooked for many years, until Dr. J. Compton-Burnett, an accomplished English homeopath, was searching for a spleen specific medicine and found his book.

In 1898, a small monograph called *Diseases of the Spleen* was published; and *Ceanothus* was adopted into the pharmacopoeia of herbalists, eclectics, homeopaths, and allopathic doctors.

Two years later, Dr. Fahnestock, did a proving of *Ceanothus* and wrote: "To my surprise the first symptom noticed was a sticking pain in the spleen, and after continued use of the remedy, there was quite an enlargement of that organ."

An actinomycete isolated from the rhizoplane of the nitrogen-fixing nodules of *C. velutinus* has been identified as a variety of *Streptomyces griseoloalbus*.

This helps give its plant signature. The S shaped roots look like an intestine and the nitrogen fixing nodules look like lymphatic mesenteric nodes.

It is a very strong antagonist against several destructive root fungal pathogens including *Phellinus, Fomes* and *Phytophthora* species. The stability and longevity of the anti-microbial substance produced by it, its consistent effect on the pathogens, its ability to colonize wood, and the ability to grow at 10 degrees Celsius, suggest it has biological control possibilities. This work, by Rose et al, was reported in the May 1980 *Canadian Journal of Microbiology*.

California Lilac (*C. thrysiflorus*) is found as far north as Victoria, BC. Natives of California including the Cahuilla believed the shrub protected them from lightning strikes by deflecting the flashes. It was known as **ISWISH**.

The micro-symbiont associated with *Ceanothus* species root is closely related to that associated with *Dryas drummondii.*

The Mexican *C. azurea* is used as a fever remedy.

MEDICINAL

CONSTITUENTS- *C. velutinus* root- ceanothic (emmolic) succinic, oxalic, malonic, malic, orthophosphoric, and pyrophosphoric acid; glutamine, glutamic acid, asparagine, aspartic acid, beta sitosterol, nonacosane, l-hexacosanol, ceanothenic acid, ceanothine, betulinic acid, betulin, octacosanoic acid, velutin, 4'-0-methyl velutin, 2-formyl-3-methoxy-A (1)-norlup-20(29)-en-28-oic acid, zizy-beranolic acid, acetyl zizyberanolic acid.
leaf- velutin. vanillic acid, tannins, syringic acid, stearic acid, phloroglucinol, para hydroxy benzoic acid, para coumaric acid, palmitic acid, n-nonacosane, myricyl alcohol, hexacosan-1-ol, gentisic acid, cinnamic acid, cerotic acid
bush- tannins (17%), velutin.
C. sanguineus root bark- cyclopeptide alkaloids, phencyclopeptines.

The roots are the important medicinal part of Redroot. They are bitter, astringent, dry and cooling. Herbalists consider it a lymphatic stimulant and tonic, useful in the treatment of tonsillitis, appendicitis, enlarged spleen or liver or wherever there is lymphatic stagnation or inflammation in the body.

When the spleen is not doing its proper job, lymph stagnates, edema results, dampness precipitates into mucous, swollen glands appear, and the blood is not adequately nourished.

The herb is useful in treating lymphatic leukemia, as well as spleen enlargement associated with hemolytic anemia.

Swollen glands, edema, pelvic congestion, enlargement and inflammation of the spleen, as well as violent shortness of breath caused by a swollen spleen, are all addressed with redroot.

Redroot is a useful herb in bronchitis with profuse mucous production and the associated pain in the liver or back.

It can be combined with other herbs for loss of appetite, general weakness, pain and weakness around the belly button, anemia, constant urging to urinate, or profuse menstruation, nosebleeds, and bleeding hemorrhoids.

It will help with lung conditions such as ruptured capillaries associated with heavy coughing.

Ovarian cysts, and other shrinking non-fibrous cysts are more easily cured when redroot is added to the formula. I have found it a useful addition in certain inflamed prostate conditions.

Chemical constituents are found in the leaves and roots, the root being stronger in action.

Other alkaloids of some varieties have been shown clinically to lower blood pressure.

From the Chinese perspective, the name “spleen” is the whole digestive-lymphatic system. Spleen yang deficiency is a condition where the heat and power of the spleen, to transport and transform fluids is so low that they stagnate. Dampness builds up, heat disappears and coldness sets in. Kapha and phlegmatic tendencies present themselves.

Chronic symptoms are cold extremities, a slow, frail pulse, watery stools containing digested food, and abdominal pain.

Previous to this a damp heat invades the whole system, and this is where the cooling and relaxant effect of Redroot comes to the fore.

In any acute inflammation with swelling of the abdomen, spleen, liver and lymphatic, think of this remedy.

When white blood cells kill bacteria and viruses, they throw debris to the lymphatic system to clear. If lymph is flowing well, there will be less congestion and healing is greatly enhanced.

The tongue, according to Matthew Wood, is enlarged, with a dirty, slick yellow, gray, white coating.

From a holistic perspective, the lymphatic system includes stagnation of fluids, precipitation of turbid lymph into mucous, poor nutrition of the blood, and tissues.

Red root is useful, as part of a constitutional formula, for those who had their tonsils or appendix removed at an early age.

It is useful for reducing risk of cancer metastasizing to lymph glands, and treating fibrocystic breasts, according to Darcy Williamson, an accomplished Idaho herbalist.

It combines well with cleavers for fibrocystic breasts, or with chasteberry for uterine fibroids.

Michael Moore mixed some of his blood with red root juice and put it under a microscope. He was able to demonstrate that *Ceanothus* acts on the electrical charge that separates the red blood cells and blood proteins from the artery wall.

This charge enhances the ability of the vessels to keep the blood cells inside them, while allowing easy transport of lymph through the sieve-like arteries. The result is the blood is better able to receive and give nutrition, and the lymph is better able to receive and remove waste.

"Think of Redroot as turning 50-weight blood (suitable only for a 1968 Chevy with a cracked block) into 10-40 weight blood. This gives Redroot a variety of tonic application: I have only scratched the surface.

It is an excellent home remedy for menstrual hemorrhage, nosebleeds, bleeding hemorrhoids, and old ulcers, as well as capillary ruptures from vomiting or coughing."

Michael continues, "for those that use oriental diagnostic methods, a rounded tablespoon of red root and a scant teaspoon of vervain brewed similarly and drunk for several days will help clear the meridians of the torso, pelvis and legs. If these are longstanding blockages and the meridians either over or under sensitive, this treatment will help to clarify diagnosis and subsequent therapy, be it acupuncture, reflexology, chiropractic or whatever."

Practitioners of TCM will find it useful in formulas that treat accumulations of blood from Qi stagnation, damp stagnation or heat, according to Thomas Garran.

The Eclectics looked at symptoms such as enlarged spleen, with a dirty white or yellow coating on tongue, and the skin is full, sallow and doughy, with an expression-less face.

In my own clinical practice, I have seen it work time and again for mononucleosis, helping the spleen reduce in swelling and inflammation. It appears to reduce in teenagers, the period of weakness and fatigue, from six months, to four to six weeks, and combines well with milk thistle seed.

It is a specific for increasing platelet counts that may have dropped due to drug therapy.

Lymphatic congestion of the intestinal tract may benefit, combining well with ocotillo bark.

Consider its use for capillary fragility or for hemolytic anemia; the latter at doses of 15-30 drops three times daily.

Consider redroot for mononucleosis, malaria, thalassemia, sickle cell anemia, recurrent tuberculosis, non-Hodgkin's lymphoma or liver or spleen enlargements caused by ciprofoxatine or related drugs. Thrombocytopenia after chemotherapy is another use for the herb. For sickle cell anemia, combine with prickly ash.

Use for chronic dry coughs, recovery from pneumonia, and in cases of interstitial cystitis associated with cold, damp congestion.

It may be useful topically as a wash for seborrheic dermatitis or psoriasis.

The dried leaf decoctions help soothe an upset stomach, mild recurring hepatitis, as well as a good gargle for sore throats or tonsillitis.

Redroot (*C. americanus*) has been researched for antimicrobial activity. Li et al, *Phytochemistry* 46:1 reported various compounds in redroot inhibit various oral pathogens, leading perhaps to another use of the herb.

Dr. Bastyr recommended the root for lymphatic leukemia, something echoed by William Mitchell. He tells of an 80 year old man who died ten years after a diagnosis of leukemia. He took 60 drops twice daily of *C. americanus* tincture.

Ceanothic acid, present in *C. velutinus*, has been found to inhibit *Streptococcus mutans, Actinomyces viscosus, Porphyromonas gingivalis* and *Prevotella intermedia.*

The first two organisms mentioned are bacteria associated with gum disease, gingivitis, and pyorrhea.

Zizyberanolic and its acetyl acid have been shown active against *Bacillus subtilis* and *Staphylococcus aureus.* The plant ash is rich in potassium, calcium, magnesium, aluminum, iron and silicon, according to Clare Goodrick-Clarke.

Work by McCutcheon et al, *J Ethnopharm* 1994 44 & 1992 37 found branches of *C. velutinus* inhibited seven of nine fungi and seven of eleven bacteria species tested.

It appears to enhance production of T cells, even in AIDS patients, but caution is noted.

Redroot reduces heavy menstrual bleeding, and is a reasonably effective coagulant and hemostat. Up to 10-15 ml may be necessary.

One study of 3.5-7 ml found the lower dose accelerated blood clotting within twenty minutes. The higher dose resulted in coagulation decreasing after one hour.

Peter Holmes, in his excellent book, *The Energetics of Western Herbs* compares redroot bark to the leaf of oriental thuja (see Cedar) in that both stop uterine bleeding, and remove blood congestion. But that is where any similarity ends.

California wild lilac (*C. thyrsiflorus*) is rich in saponins, and the flowers and fruit produce a nice soap.

Ellingwood reported on findings of Henderson who chewed some berries that relieved his sore, dry and constricted throat.

"He determined to try them in other cases of throat disease and had a tincture prepared from the berries. Shortly after, in a severe epidemic of malignant diphtheria, he treated eighteen cases without the loss of one, using the Ceanothus in all cases. He has used it since in diphtheria, pharyngitis, tonsillitis and nasal catarrh with good results. He gives it in diseases of the mucous surface where the discharge is profuse, thick ane tenacious. For a gargle he used two drams of tincture to four ounces of water. It foams in the throat like the peroxide of hydrogen and must be used with care…He believes the berries should be gathered just before they are ripe, to obtain the best action."

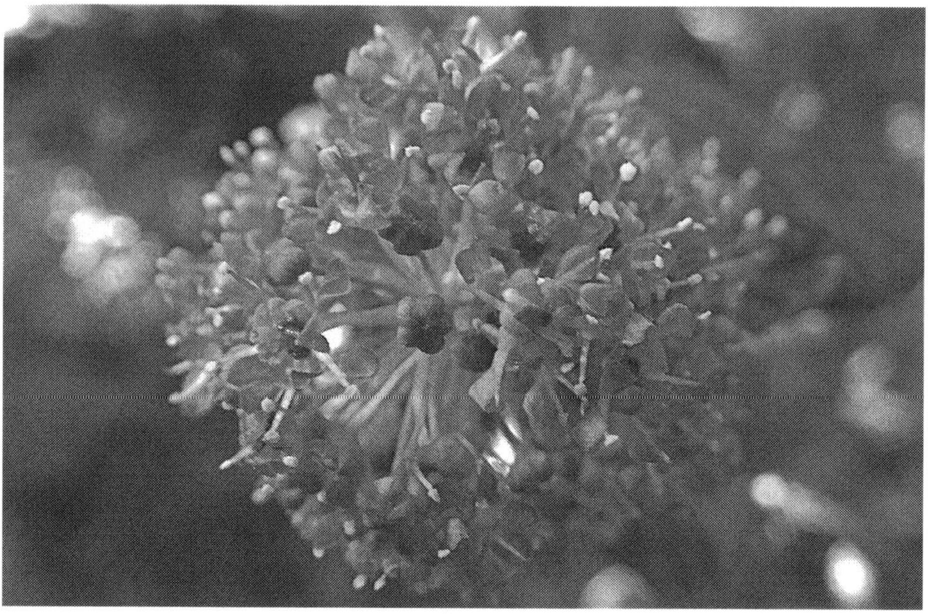

California Lilac (*C. thyrsiflorus*) flower

HOMEOPATHY

Ceanothus seems to possess a specific relation to the spleen. It is generally a left-sided remedy, for anemic patients where liver and spleen are at fault.

It is for enlargement of the spleen, chronic bronchitis with profuse secretions, profuse menses, and yellow weakening leucorrhea. There is a constant urging to urinate, and may contain bile and sugar, appearing green and frothy.

DOSE- First to third potency. The mother tincture is prepared from the dried leaves of Ceanothus species. Use 6X potency for thalassemia. Proving by Fahnestock with two male provers and tincture in 1899. Clinical symptoms improved in a 42 year old male diagnosed with non-Hodgkin's lymphoma, follicular, mixed type, stage III by Eric Sommermann with Ceanothus 12C potency.

California Lilac (*C. thrysiflorus*) is for pharyngitis, tonsillitis, nasal catarrh.

DOSE- Tincture internally and as a gargle. This plant grows all over Victoria BC and surrounding area.

PLANT WAX

C. velutinus contains ceryl and myricyl alcohols, palmitic, stearic and cerotic acid, hydrocarbons and resins, beta amyrin, and ursolic acid.

The leaves of the dried bush can be ground, sifted and extracted with gasoline or any other suitable solvent. There is wax yield of 7.3%, with a dark olive-green colour, that is hard and brittle.

It melts at 78 degrees Celsius, has specific gravity of 0.988, saponification number of 93.4 and iodine number of 19.3. After treatment with fuller's earth, the crude wax is dark yellow. The resins have a distinctive terpene odour.

ESSENTIAL OIL

The essential oil from leaves contains cinnamic acid ethyl esters, cinnamyl cinnamate, paracoumaric acid, and salicyaldehydes.

FLOWER ESSENCE

Deerbrush (*C. integerrimus*) flower essence is for mixed or conflicting motives, where subconscious feelings propel outer actions.

The positive qualities from its use are gentle purity, clarity of purpose, and sincerity of motive. **FLOWER ESSENCE SOCIETY**

SPIRITUAL PROPERTIES

According to traditional Greek medicine, the emotion connected with the spleen is melancholia. The word "melancholia" means black bile and refers to a substance which is supposed to be stored in the spleen. An excess of "black bile" or "melancholia" causes the corresponding emotion.

The Chinese attribute the same psychological disorder to the spleen.

In ancient Chinese medicine it was stated that the spleen "stores the ideas", or images. Excessive thought, brooding and introspection is an imbalance associated with the spleen. This turns to pensiveness, brooding and melancholia.

The word melancholy is not well understood at the present time. Generally, we use the word "depression". Actually, these two words do not mean exactly the same thing.

Melancholy is associated with a lack of direction, purpose, creativity, with an artistic funk or an inability to think oneself out of a predicament. Depression, while it may include this, is more often associated with grief and loss.

The psychological faculty most closely associated with the spleen is the imagination. Images flit to and fro through our imagination, sort of like the particles circulating in the lymphatic fluids. An image comes to rest from time to time, alighting on some filament of consciousness and arising into our everyday awareness, just as a particle of nutriment comes to the cell that needs it and is absorbed within.

When the spleen is strong, the imagination flourishes. Life is happy, well-adjusted, vibrant, and meaningful. This is an important organ indeed. **WOOD**

PERSONALITY TRAITS

There is melancholy and purposelessness in the spleen patient. He may become rigid in his outlook and lose his sense of humor, growing melancholy and moralistic.

In a negative state, responsibility—the negative pole of the idealism that shows in the healthy person—hangs heavily. They are over responsible and fastidious; life wearies them with its perceived demands.

On a psychological level, they experience stagnancy—lack of drive, lack of ambition. The individual may feel he has more to do in life, but he does not know what to be at. He goes on with the same job, unable to break free, but all the time he frets that his life is passing without his having achieved much.

Ambitions that have seemed important in the past now seem to have served their turn.

The individual wants something new, but does not know what. Everything that might appeal to him seems out of reach—too little money, too little time. **GOODRICK-CLARKE**

For those who do not have access to beaver musk, I recommend **EGISH GIGESHEPITA HISHA**, elkweed, for serious lover seekers. Just rub some of the dried leaves on your hands, rub a bit on the person you want to attract and walk away. Someone will follow you, I guarantee it. Sometimes a honeymoon follows too.

Elkweed (*Ceanothus velutinus*), sometimes called red root, is a short bush that grows in wet places in the mountains west of here. A sprig of its dried leaves can work wonders. It is strong, potent. We should call it "obsession". People become obsessed with you when you wear it.

We have fun with that elkweed. You can smell it all over at some powwows. Elk love it too, in case you were wondering. They nibble on the blossoms, and it just drives them crazy. **SNELL**

BOTANICA POETICA

Redroot
(*Ceanothus americanus* & *C. velutinus*)
If mono has its grip on you
I think I know what you could do
When your spleen is quite enlarged
And your liver is engorged
We have an herb that filters blood
Helps the drainage, clears the mud
Lymphatics it will stimulate
Congestion, it eliminates
If you've overdone the fats
You have a headache due to that
Here's the one to rid the waste
Ceanothus Americanus, take in haste
It's astringent, it's a filter
When your system's out of kilter
Take Red Root to cleanse and clear
Watch your swelling disappear!
SYLVIA CHATROUX MD

ASTROLOGY

Saturn is Chronos, the god of time who rules entropy, limitation, aging, and decay. A negative Saturn condition is seen in the premature aging and running down of the energy of the patient. The hair may go gray or start falling out.

The physical degeneration of someone with spleen and liver problems will be quite marked, with weakness, stiffness, and pessimism. Without correction, there can be a continual slide to chronic disease, cancer, rheumatism, and other such Saturnine diseases. Under a positive corrective remedy the spleen regains its powers of separating wastes, which enables the body to regain control of its self-healing capacities—and the lymphatic system is key in this. The positive side of Saturn is the structuring and organizing principle that can reestablish order, correct elimination function, adjust mineral metabolism, and bring poise and optimism.

C. GOODRICK-CLARKE

RECIPES

COLD INFUSION- 2-4 ounces, as needed. One part to 32 parts water. Steep overnight and bring to warm temperature without boiling.

DECOCTION- 2 tbsp of dried root simmered in one quart of water for twenty minutes. Refrigerate. Take 10-12 ounces three times daily an hour before each meal.

TINCTURE- 20-40 drops 3x daily in ice cold water. Tincture is prepared from fresh root at 1:2 at 95% or dry at 1:5 in 50% alcohol. Gather fresh root and stem bark in early spring, before flowering. Root/root bark should be pink to red. Cut the fresh roots immediately before they harden like rocks.

What's with the cold? When taken cold on an empty stomach, the herbal action is better sited in the lymphatic tissue. If taken warm or hot, there would be more diaphoretic or sweating action that may exacerbate a skin condition, and would not help at the deeper, lymphatic levels.

Matthew Wood notes that material doses can cause aggravations, such as swollen tongue in some individuals.

CAUTION- For those allergic to aspirin, or with blood disorders, use care with red root. Do not use at the same time as anti-coagulants.

Use with caution in hypotension, as blood pressure can be lowered in some individuals.

It should be used in moderation during pregnancy, and those with diarrhea/loose stool. Use caution with dosage in acute spleen inflammation. Do not take two weeks prior to surgery or following surge of blood.

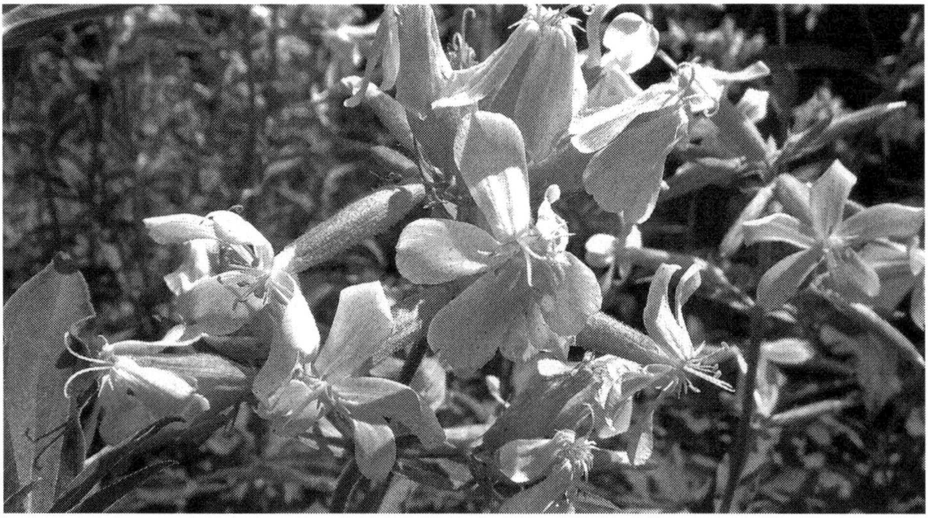

Soapwort

SOAPWORT
BOUNCING BET
(*Saponaria officinalis* L.)
(*Lychnis saponaria*)
COW COCKLE
COW SOAPWORT
FORBIDDEN PALACE FLOWER
(*S. vaccaria* L.)
(*Vaccaria pyramidata*)
(*V. segatalis*)
(*V. hispanica* [Mill.] Raushert)
ROCK SOAPWORT
(*S. ocymoides* L.)
PART USED- root, flower, leaf, seed

Saponaria is from the Latin **SAPO** meaning soap and **ARIA** meaning like or similar to. Bouncing Bet, another common name, comes from the use of the plant to clean beer bottles by barmaids (generally called Bet or Betsy).

What bounced is less certain! Another likely origin is the similarity of the inflated calyx and scalloped leaves to the jiggling rear view of a laundress. Bet is a version of Betty, an older term for a laundress.

Since the name arose in England during Elizabethan times, the name Bet could be in her honour.

Vaccaria is related to its early use as a forage plant for cows.

An early Greek name **CATHARSIS**, meaning a cleanser or purifier, referred to both the soapy uses and purgative effect on the body used medicinally.

The Romans called it Herba Lanaria, or Wool Herb, using it to clean wool before weaving it into cloth.

Soapwort is a naturalized perennial on the prairies, frequently found in sunny fields and along railways. It is native to western Asia, but was grown in European gardens for centuries for medicine and soap. The plant has no smell in daytime, but at night exudes a delicate violet-clove like scent for attracting moths. Cow Cockle is an introduced annual, with no scent in their pale pink flowers.

As far back as Dioscorides, the plant has been attributed with curing liver, coughs and kidney stones. At that time it was known as **STRUTHION**.

Anglo-Saxons used the plant for liver complaints and bladder stones by adding it to beer. Leprosy was treated with application of the crushed plant mixed with whole meal and vinegar. And for general swellings the plant was crushed along with barley and wine.

The Assyrians made soap from the plant back in the eighth century B.C. And in the Middle Ages, the plant was known as **HERBA FULLONIS**, since fullers used the leaves to clean cloth. In France, the plant is still known as *Herbe a Foulon*. In Switzerland, sheep were washed with a mixture of roots, leaves and water before they were shorn.

Even today, with the wide range of synthetic detergents and cleansers available, soapwort is the first choice for conservators of antique fabrics, furniture and picture cleaning. It has a beneficial action on the proteins of silk and wool, and is used to restore colour and sheen to old and faded fabrics, ancient tapestries, embroideries and brocades.

Its saponins efficiently and harmlessly return an original luster to delicate china and precious glass (see recipes below).

It is still cultivated in Syria today for washing woolens.

Early Pennsylvania Dutch used the plant not only for cleansing, but to add a foamy head to their beers, a tradition brought from Europe.

Culpepper called soapwort "an absolute cure in the French pox (syphilis)", a usage recounted by Mrs. Grieve in her famous book. He adds "how true it is, I leave others to judge". Well, no judgment but we know it does not.

It has been used traditionally for gout, liver problems, rheumatism, skin disease, constipation, bronchial congestion and as a diuretic.

In India, a specially prepared root is used to increase mother's milk.

After its introduction to the New World, various native tribes began to use the plant medicinally. The Cherokee made a poultice of root for boils, and Mahuna used the root juice as a hair tonic, and applied leaf poultices over spleen pain.

In Mexico, and elsewhere, the cut plant is kept in a bowl inside the house, to discourage the flies.

The movie industry uses the surfactant properties of Soapwort to keep their film clean during manufacture.

Soapwort helps detoxify and break down trinitroluene (TNT).

Cow cockle, the annual, is used today in Pakistan for jaundice, rheumatism, hepatic eruptions, and venereal ulcers.

The saponins from the roots are very irritating to the digestive system. Livestock eating hay containing seeds may be poisoned. And the leaf and root will poison fish when put in pond water.

Externally, the juice from leaves and root can be used for skin itching related to poison ivy, acne, eczema, psoriasis, and drawing boils. In Italy, a fomentation is made from the roots to soothe itching caused by dermatosis.

Root decoctions or fomentations help remove discoloration from bruises or black eyes.

In China, the reddish mustard-like seeds are used for point plaster therapy- that is, they are taped on specific acupuncture points for a length of time to treat addictions, etc.

The herb goes by several names including, **CHIN KUNG HUA**, Forbidden Palace Flower, and **CHIN CHIEN YEN-T'AI**, meaning golden lamp on silver pedestal.

In Japan, it is used traditionally to activate blood flow and promote milk production.

The de-hulled seeds of Cow Cockle contain over 77% starch, and may find application in food, as a low fat cream substitute, and in cosmetic industries. It has a protein component useful as a feed supplement and/or production of ribosome inactivating proteins for medicinal use.

The saponin content may be useful as a substitute for quillaja saponins, and the cyclo-peptides are useful medicinal compounds.

The seed is the same shape and size as canola, indicating that no equipment changes would be needed. Its addition to birdseed mixes has contributed to its wide spread dispersal.

Dr. John Balsevich at the *Plant Biotechnology Institute* in Saskatoon is investigating and isolating individual saponins and working on developing elite germplasm to produce high concentrations of quillaja type saponins. These saponins are presently extracted from Soap Bark (*Quillaja saponaria*) with one thousand tons required to produce 180-200 tons of crude extract.

Soap Bark saponins are used as adjuvants in immunostimulating complex vaccine, where they enhance the antibody response to any antigen. Bomford, *Phytother Res* 1988 2. At the present time they are more widely used in veterinary, than human medicine.

Rock Soapwort (*S. ocymoides*) is often planted in rock gardens, in well-drained soil with full sun. It is a hardy perennial often preferred by gardeners who find the *S. officinalis* too weedy looking. I do not have the data, but feel certain that it contains similar constituents to the others.

Soapwort is difficult to propagate from seed, with better results from established cuttings. Do not plant near fishponds as drainage may cause toxicity.

MEDICINAL

CONSTITUENTS- *S. officinalis*- seed saponins (up to 5%, including saporubrin and saporubrinic acid) sapotoxin, saporin, spinasterol, quillaic acid, genin, gums, mucilage, resins, flavonoids like saponarin and vitexin; vitamin C, oxalic acid. root- saponins, water soluble polysaccharides (15.7%) composed mainly of 16.09 galactose, 6.7 glucose and 1.17 arabinose.
S. vaccaria- seed- kaempferol, sapxanthone, vaccarin, vaccariose; vaccaroside E, G, and H; segetoside I, segetalins A&B, various saponins (vacsegosides, gypsogenin, isosaponarin, saponaretin, vitexin), glucuronic acid, glucose, arabinose, xylose, protein (15-16%), starch (60%), lipids. The seeds contain an abundance of both macro and micro-minerals. The seed is richest in arginine, aspartic and glutamic acids; and four times the lysine of wheat.

Soapwort roots, due largely to saponins, are an effective expectorant for dry coughs and bronchitis. It has a detergent-like effective on gallstones, and increases bile flow.

It is a powerful laxative, with purgative and griping action when taken in large doses, however.

Externally, the root decoctions can be used as a wash for eczema and other related skin problems, including psoriasis, acne, poison ivy and boils. Small amounts of the tea, at body temperature, can be used in conjunction.

Soapwort is a pelvic venous decongestant, especially useful to women with congestive dysmenorrhea.

As Peter Holmes says, “The remedy succeeds best in individuals suffering from chronic forms of eczema and swollen glands with underlying kidney and liver deficiency- especially when they complain of always feeling tired and run down”.

Cebo et al, *Herba Polonica* 1976 22 reported that saponin extracts of soapwort have analgesic properties.

Soapwort seeds contain a protein (0.4% of total seed weight), or 7% of the total seed protein with exciting potential. Studies conducted by Stirpe et al in Italy (1983) showed the protein actually inhibited protein synthesis (ribosome inactivating); as well as anti-viral activity.

Saporin has unusual stability, and is a suitable candidate for various biotechnological applications.

Italian studies by Santanche et al, found saporin showed marked resistance to denaturation by urea, guanidine and proteolysis.

Soapwort is both an alterative with restorative qualities, as well as a lymphatic and liver detoxifier with powerful laxative and anti-tumour effects.

The saponins have shown to be powerful cytotoxic agents *in vitro*, when conjugated to molecular targeting anti-bodies or protein ligands; including human lymphoma, leukemia, melanoma and breast cancer cells. Teece et al, *Melanoma Research* 1991; Siena et al, *Cancer Research* 1989.

A more recent study by Balsevich et al, *Fitoterapia* 83:1 found purified segetoside H & I active against breast and prostate cancer cell lines. The total extract was most active against colon cancer lines.

Gasperi-Campani et al, *Experimental Hematology* 1989, suggested a root extract, saporin 6, inhibited tumour growth, particularly leukemic cells.

Saporin shows activity against *Candida albicans* ribosomes. Park et al, *Planta Medica* 2002 216:2.

Anti-virus activity of an herbal preparation containing Soapwort roots, Black Elderberry flowers and the leaves and flowers of St. John's Wort was tested in Bulgaria in 1996. The preparation, named SHS-174, inhibited the reproduction of strain specific viruses. Serkedjieva et al, *Phyto Res* 1990 4:3.

Extracts of the root show activity against gram positive and negative bacteria.

The leaves contain similar constituents but are weaker.

Arabinoglucogalactan polysaccharides in the root have general biological interest for the immune system.

Cow cockle has several constituents of interest. Kaempferol, isolated from the callus culture was administered to lab rats orally. Kumar et al, in 1989. It was found to inhibit the production of sperm, thereby affecting fertility.

In neighboring Pakistan, Kazmi et al, in the same year, isolated sapxanthone, from the plant. Malik et al, in the next year isolated a novel oligosaccharide from the plant called vaccariose.

Cow cockle seed is used in China, under the Mandarin **JIN GONG HUA**, or **WANG BU LIU XING**; or the Cantonese **WONG BO LAU CHIN**. It is prepared as a decoction, or tincture. Wang Bu Liu means literally, "the king does not linger", suggesting movement without stopping.

I have found it called **CHIN-CHIEN YEN-T'AI**, or Golden Lamp on Silver Pedestal; and **CHIN KUNG HUA**, Forbidden Palace Flower, in various books.

The alcohol extraction strongly promotes menstruation. Cow cockle seed can be used as a uterine stimulant in cases of amenorrhea, prolonged pregnancy, or stalled labour and of course, is contraindicated in pregnancy. For dysmenorrhea and amenorrhea combine with Safflower petals.

It may, however, be used in cases of insufficient or absent lactation; or cases of breast infection like mastitis.

There is a saying among the working people of China. "When women take Wang Biu Liu Xing, their breasts grow and flow with milk."

The uncooked seed is often combined with Forsythia fruit and Dandelion leaf and root for acute mastitis, or inflamed breasts.

The stir-fried seed is used for amenorrhea or oligomenorrhea due to lower abdominal blood stasis, retention of fetus, or strangury with blood, painful urination with urgency.

Two cyclic peptides, segetalin A and B exhibit estrogen-like activity; and increase effects of oxytocin on the uterus. *Planta Medica* 1995 61:6 561-2.

It is a specific in cases of benign prostate congestion, often added to a patent formula called Prostate Gland Pills. It works well but during the treatment it causes some men to lose erections, a side effect that disappears after use of the herb. However, men with prostate pain and inflammation should refrain from intercourse, so it all works out.

The influence on both male and female reproductive systems may be due, in part to the cyclic pentapeptides, segatalins. These compounds, found in the seed, possess estrogen-like activity.

HJ Zhang et al, *J Ethnopharmacology* 2012 Nov 29 found extracts useful for prevention and treatment of benign prostatic hypertrophy.

Segetalins have been found to possess significant anti-tumour activity. Itokawa, *J Biochem Mol Biol Biophysics* 2000 4:3.

The seeds ameliorate osteopenia by inhibition of bone resorption. Shih et al, *J Nat Med* 63:4.

For the treatment of herpes, including herpes zoster (shingles), the seeds are toasted, powdered, mixed in oil, and applied externally to affected area.

For ulcers, boils, painful swellings and wounds, a simple wash is prepared by decoction. For more serious abscesses of the breasts, testes or lymphadenitis, the washes are administered frequently.

Recent studies published in the *British Journal of Cancer* by Di Massimo et al looked at ribosome inactivating proteins from *V. pyramidata*.

The saponins and alkaloids from seeds have been found effective against Erhlich ascites, breast and hepatoma cancer cell lines.

Balsevich et al, *Fitoterapia* 2012 83:1 found bi-desmosidic saponins in seeds active against breast and prostate cancer cell lines.

The study showed the seed extract inhibited growth of grafted human tumour cells in nude mice experiments.

HOMEOPATHY

Saponaria is used where there is an indifferent, apathetic temperament, and also in depressive states with sleeplessness, and when there are stabbing pains above the eye sockets, worse on the left side, on movement, and towards evening. There may also be a throbbing above the eyes with congestion of blood in the head and a feeling of weariness in the neck, prickling in the eyeballs, ciliary neuralgia, photophobia and increased intraocular pressure.

The symptoms might make us think of Saponaria in the kind of preliminary stages or complaints found in glaucoma.

Difficulty in swallowing, nausea, heartburn, and a sensation of fullness in the stomach is not relieved by eructation.

Palpitations with a slow pulse and anxiety states may be an indication for Saponaria, whilst otherwise it is almost exclusively used in the treatment of acute colds, coryza, and throat pains, tonsillitis, pharyngitis, and laryngitis.

In combination remedies, Saponaria is used because of its blood cleansing action. It facilitates that elimination of homotoxins which have been freed through harmless catarrhal symptoms such as an acute cold or in serious cases like tonsillitis. Saponaria then compensates for this by inhibiting inflammation in a biological way by changing the homotoxic terrain.

DOSE- Tincture to low potencies.

The mother tincture is prepared from the dried root. Proving by Shier with 26 provers with tincture, 1x, 2x, 3x, 6x, and 10x in 1901. Additions by Boericke.

Saponium is for mind cross and unsettled upon waking in morning. Food tastes wrong, indifference to all around, aphasia-like conditions, troubled by difficulty remembering common words.

Desire to be left alone from beginning to end of menses. Dreams of urinating.

Oysters cause gastrointestinal distress. Crops of boils, very angry and ugly.

DOSE- First to 30th potency. Saponinum is a glycoside saponin from root. First proving by Hill with seven females and ten males at 1x, 2x, 3x, 12x, 30x in 1874.

SEED OIL

The seeds of Cow cockle (*S. vaccaria*) contain about 4% oil composed of unusual composition. This includes D-pinitol, vaccarin, vaccaxanthone, segetoside, vaccegosides A, B, C and D, and 1,8-dihydroxy-3, 5-dimethoxy-9H-xanthen-9-one.

Triglycerides compose over 70% of the lipid total, with phosphatydl serine at 3.1%. and phosphatydl choline at 9.7%.

The major fatty acids are linoleic, oleic and palmitic acids. D-pinitol has application in high blood sugar.

HYDROSOL

Viaud suggests that soapwort hydrosol is of benefit in treating eczema, furuncles and diabetes.

Soapwort water is prepared from the herb and root in June. It is used for skin abscesses, strains about the breast, and pestilence.

BRUNSCHWIG

FLOWER ESSENCES

Soapwort (*S. ocymoides*) flower essence is for use where there is bewilderment and lack of vision. For the "What the Hell am I doing here?" type of feeling.

This is a stage frequently encountered during personal development as the older identities lose their grip. In the vacuum that is then created, there is the need for a quiet healing space in life.

This remedy is to help those at this point in their lives, also helping them to distance themselves from previous attitudes to life that could adversely affect them. **BAILEY**

Bouncing Bet flower essence is for those who feel out of balance and disharmony with self or with their partner; feel closed down sexually, have trouble loving themselves, or feel disassociated from others.

LIVING FLOWER

SPIRITUAL PROPERTIES

Bouncing Bet, or Saponaria is related to the right use of the granted grace. No deformation, no diminution, no exaggeration- a clear sincerity. **THE MOTHER**

DOCTRINE OF SIGNATURES

The smooth leaves grow in pairs and the soft petals have two parts, representing balance, union, and harmony. The sensuality of the plant and is expression of male/female, penis/vulva, also represents balance and the awakening of sexual energy rising up the spine as the kundalini force and spiraling up to the heart.

The pale pink and creamy lavender colors represent the heart chakra, radiating compassion, oneness, bliss and love. **PALLASDOWNEY**

RECIPES

SOAPWORT TINCTURE- 20-40 drops 3 times daily. Make the tincture from the whole dried plant at 1:5 and 60% alcohol.

SOAPWORT DECOCTION- Soak four tbsp of dried root or half that of fresh in one litre of cold water for five hours. Bring to boil and simmer for ten minutes. Drink 2-4 oz up to 4 times daily. Daily dose is 10-15 grams.

CAUTION- Avoid soapwort if there are ulcers or severe gastrointestinal disorders. Avoid during pregnancy, due to both uterine stimulation and laxative effect.

Do not take during indigestion or diarrhea associated with cold or damp conditions of the intestines, or cold, damp phlegm conditions of the lungs.

COW COCKLE SEED- decoct 5-7 grams in two doses, between meals. It is extremely bitter, and often combined with other herbs.

Cow cockle seed is not recommended during pregnancy, or in patients without blood vessel integrity.

SOAP- Take a large cheesecloth or muslin bagful of soapwort leaves, chopped and bruised, with about a half pint of water. Boil together for a half hour, then strain off the soapy liquid. It leaves a slight green stain that rinses out.

Or, take one oz. of the crushed dried root, and put it in a pot with 8 cups of cold water. Bring to a boil, and simmer 20 minutes. Cool and strain.

Store either in fridge for up to one month. Some authors suggest the root cannot be simmered, as this will inactivate the final product. Not true.

Note- If embroidery or tapestry on canvas is to be treated, it should be prepared before washing so that immediately after, it can be fixed on a stretcher to restore its original shape. To do this, merely sew strips of material all around the piece to square the shape and have a stretcher of 4 pieces of strong wood ready to use. Then, right after washing, drive thumbtacks through the new material onto the stretcher.

STILLINGIA
QUEEN'S ROOT
QUEEN'S DELIGHT
(*Stillingia sylvatica* L.)
(*Sapium sylvaticum* [L.] Torr.)
PARTS USED- root

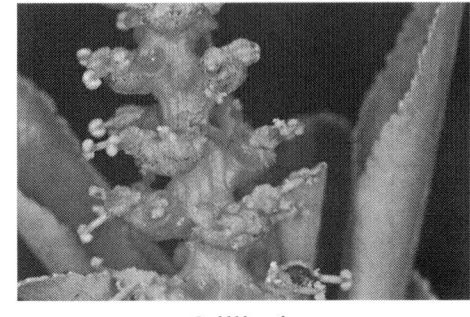

Stillingia
(Courtesy of John Gwaltney)

Stillingia is named after the 18th century author and botanist, Benjamin Stillingfleet.

The perennial plant is found from Maryland to the Gulf coast of Louisiana, on sandy soil and pine barrens.

Vermeulen contributes. "The Seminole Indians employed Stillingia for two types of disease. They used it for 'bird' sickness with diarrhoea, vomiting and appetite loss and also for menstruation sickness with yellow eyes and skin, weakness and shaking head. Particularly in the southern U.S., the queen's root once had a considerable reputation in domestic, regular and eclectic medical practice. The drug emerged in the 18th century as a treatment for yaws, an ailment common among slaves, characterized by infection of skin, bones, joints and caused by the spirochete *Treponema pallidum* subsp. *pertenue*. In homeopathy, the yaws nosode is known as Framboesinum. Although serologically and morphologically indistinguishable from *Treponema pallidum,* the spirochete associated with syphilis, *T. pertenue* differs from the former in tis non-venereal transmission and in its clinical manifestations."

Dr. King noted. "When the specific indications for the drug have followed the results have been fully as good as have been obtained from any of the anti-syphilitics. The case for its exhibition in syphilitic and other affections are those in which the tissues are feeble and are tardily removed and renewed; the mucous membranes are predominantly affected and the skin secondarily; and the mucous membranes are tumid, red and glistening, and secretion is scanty".

MEDICINAL

CONSTITUENTS- various diterpene esters including phorbol, ingenane and daphnane, 10-12% tannins, up to 3.25% essential oil, fatty oils, resins, alkaloids including stillingine, gums, starch.

The root was official in the *US Pharmacopoeia* from 1842 to 1916. In the 19th century it was used as a deep-acting alterative and blood cleanser for syphilitic miasm. Later Eclectic physicians like Felter thought overwise.

"We do not believe it is anti-syphilitic, but is one of the best alteratives that can be exhibited in syphilitic and strumous cachexias, greatly aiding other and more powerful agents, as the iodide of potassium. In all phases of secondary syphilis—cutaneous syphilides, mucous patches, ulcers and periosteal pain and nodular and glandular enlargements—it renders good auxilary service through its depurative action…It is one of the most effectual drugs we have ever used for the irritable winter cough of the middle-aged and old. Stillingia may be used in chronic periosteal rheumatism, so-called, of unproved origin, but probably syphilitic; and in skin diseases having a remote syphilitic history."

Scudder wrote that the herb "increases waste and excretion, but its principal action probably is upon the lymphatic system, favoring the formation of good lymph, hence good blood and nutrition."

The root is bitter, pungent, cool and dry helping to clear damp cold, lymphadenitis, eczema and liver stagnation. Skin itching with pruritis and chronic weeping and wet discharge may be helped.

Osteoma (bony tumor) of the head, face and tibia, including periosteum is relieved.

Inflammations of a chronic nature including arthritis, lymphangitis and dermatitis are soothed and cleared.

I used this herb successfully many years ago on a young eight year old girl with egg-sized bony tumors on legs below knees. It took several months for the protrusions to soften, reduce and disappear.

In fact, stillingia is the "go to" herb when it comes to bone cancer.

Throat inflammation of a chronic nature, especiallly with dry heat and hoarseness is helped, due in part to essential oil conent. This makes it useful for chronic and acute laryngitis and pharyngitis. According to King, the sedative action addresses "irritative disorders of the fauces, trachea and bronchiae". It was very popular in the 19th century for croup, a barky, hoarse dry cough, viral in nature.

Liver congestion with fatigue, associated with swollen glands may respond well.

Matthew Wood suggests combining it with burdock root for chronic furunculosis.

HOMEOPATHY

Depression of spirits and gloomy forebodings. Aversion to doing anything, remorse and wanting to go where one is not annoyed.

Sweating, sensations of scalding, burning, dryness and smarting. Sharp, darting pains, with chronic rheumatism, syphilitic periosteal rhematism. Cold on going to bed and then breaking out in sweat. Has lost all strength and energy.

Heavy pressure on front of brain, or feeling brain is too large for skull. Ball or lump in throat. Bones of elbow sore and about to separate. Salty taste in mouth.

Bony tumors on head and face. White stools resembling curds. Excess itching below knees, without eruption. Worse from cold, better from warmth and bed.

DOSE- Tincture to third potency. Self experiments by Nichols with tincture in 1865; Eckles 1866-1869; Cunningham 1967 and Ingraham with tincture in 1868. Proving by Preston with three males with tincture and third dilution in 1869; Taber with three provers with tincture and chewing fresh root in 1974; clinical observations by Hale.

RECIPES

TINCTURE- Make from freshly, dried stem 1:5 at 40% alcohol. Dosage is 2 to 4 ml daily in divided doses.

DECOCTION- Use freshly, dried stem in ratio of 1:32. Use 6-14 grams daily in divided doses. The well stored dried bark has a six month shelf life.

CAUTION- Use with caution in Yin deficient conditions. Large doses may cause nausea or loose stools.

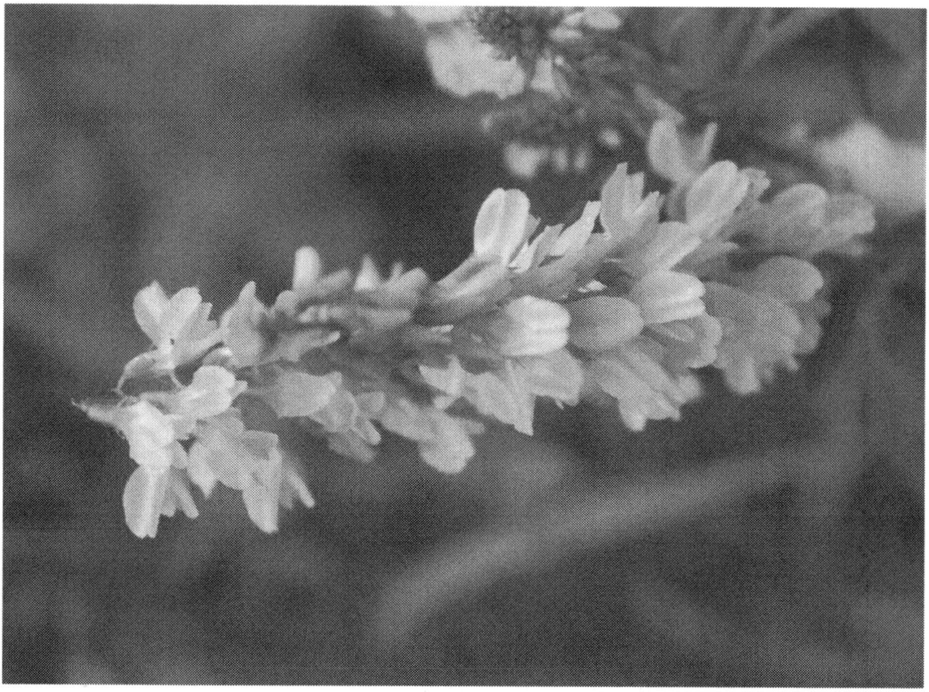

Sweet Clover

YELLOW SWEET CLOVER
SWEET CLOVER
CLOVER, SWEET YELLOW
(*Melilotus officinalis* [L.] Lam.**)**
(*M. altissimus*)
CLOVER, SWEET WHITE
(*M. alba* Medikus**)**
(*M. officinalis* subsp. *albus* [Medik.] H. Ohashi & Tateishi**)**
PARTS USED- flowers, leaves, seeds, and roots

Melilotus is from the Greek ***MEL***, meaning honey, and ***LOTUS***, after the lotus flower. ***MEL*** is also from folklore; that this plant sprung from the blood of the lion killed by Emperor Adrian.

The Yellow and White sweet clover are introduced biennials to this country, but grow abundantly in field and roadside ditches, and up to six feet tall. They sometimes flower the first year, acting like annuals, but self sow prolifically.

Generally speaking, the White Sweet Clover is taller and has more fragrant flowers.

The early Egyptians used melilot for treating earaches and intestinal worms, by drinking a tea of the leaves.

Galen treated swollen joints and dispersed tumours with Melilot plasters, (similar types can still be bought in English pharmacies), hence the former name Plaster Clover.

The dried leaves of sweet clover add a vanilla-like flavour to baked goods, snuff and tobacco. It is laid, like Labrador tea, among woolens to protect them from moths.

The seeds are coumarin-like, and according to James Duke, may be substituted for Tonka Beans, as a vanilla substitute. Duke suggests the seed tea as a cold remedy. In Pakistan, the seeds are decocted, tea is cooled, and then one-half cup is taken frequently to reduce fevers.

Traditionally, sweet clover was considered a good remedy for eyesight.

Sauer in his *Compendious Herbal*, gives a recipe for soothing the swollen privates in men. A handful of yellow clover flowers, chamomile flowers, flaxseed and faba bean flour, with a little wormwood, was boiled in milk and formed into a plaster and laid upon the affected parts.

The root was taken up in the waning of the August moon and hung on the neck.

The Irish herbalist K'Eogh reported in 1735: "A woman had a swelling for a year or more on her right side. It was cured by three or four times rubbing the grieved part with the oil made of Melilot."

In China, it was worn in the same manner for protection against unwholesome influence or burned to summon up ancestral spirits. The seed was used in bowel complaints and infantile diarrhea. Poultices of chopped plant were placed on swellings. Sweet Clover is used in TCM and known as **TSUN TS' AO**.

Unani medicine uses decoctions for inflammatory conditions of the spleen, liver, intestines, uterus and rectum.

Dicoumarol, used to kill rats and mice, is extracted from fermented melilot. Coumarin derivatives show anti-fungal activity of 100% for up to three weeks, suggesting a natural pesticide. Brooker et al, *Commun Agric Appl Biol Sci* 2007 72:4. The isoflavonoid, medicarpin is anti-fungal.

The introduced plant was not used extensively, by native people. The Slave tribe named it **DENELI NAYDI**, or Man Medicine, probably as part of a love charm. The Iroquois used infusions of white sweet clover for typhoid-like fevers caused by smelling dead snakes. They used cold infusions for colds caused by becoming chilled.

Yellow Sweet Clover was used for the Navaho for the same purpose. The Lakota call it sunstroke medicine, due to thinning of blood that relieves congestive headaches.

An old Ukrainian settlers recipe was to boil the whole white sweet clover plant with barley seeds, and drink it as a general tonic. The neighboring Poles used strained infusions as an eyewash, and in a springtime May Wine. An old folk name is **UROKOWE ZIELE**, or spell plant, indicating its use in subverting the evil eye, or bad magic.

The dried herb adds flavour to marinades, especially rabbit stew, and Gruyere cheese. The plant is prolific, producing some 350,000 seeds from one plant, and surviving in ground for over 80 years.

Dihydrocoumarin, present in Sweet Clover, is used as a flavouring agent in soft drinks, yogurt, muffins, as well as fragrance for cosmetics, lotions and soaps. It has the sweet, herbaceous scent of new mown hay and is used at up to 100 ppm in gelatins, puddings, and frozen dairy. Almost all the DHC on the market is produced by chemical synthesis, making a compound of biological origin more appealing to commercial operations.

Work by Haser et al, suggests the use of various *Saccharomyces cerevisiae, Pseudomonas orientalis,* or *Bacillus cereus* strains to convert coumarin to DHC.

MEDICINAL

CONSTITUENTS- *M. officinalis*- trans-2-hydroxycinnamic acid glucoside, bishydroxy coumarin (dicumarol), resins, dihydrocoumarin, melilotoside, 4-hydroxyphenylacetic acid, salicylic, vanillic, protochatechuic, gallic, caffeic, ferulic, melilotic and gentisic acid, isorhamnetin, hydrocoumarns including umbelliferone, scopoletin, herniarin, and fraxidin; 4-hydroxybenzoic acid, flavone pigments robinin and clovin and essential oils. Free coumarin in the dried herb is 0.4-0.9%, and is concentrated in the flower buds and fresh leaves from tips of branches. Also contains various oleanene saponins.
seeds- anti-estrogenic and anti-phlogistic effect.
M. alba- 4-hydroxycoumarin, scopoletin, melilotic acid, triterpenoid derivatives; medicarpin and melilotocarpans A,B,C,D, and E; coumaric acid, dicumaral, up to 16% protein, quercitin-3-rhamnoside, robinoside, soyasapogenol B.
Seeds–canavanin, trigonelline, dicurmol SOD, peroxidase, 8% fat, 42% protein, glucose, pentosans 8%, resins, starch; narcotic in nature.
root- saponins (1.2%)

Research into sweet clover began when an observant farmer in Wisconsin noted his cattle dying from eating it.

He contacted his local agriculture research station, and they found coumarin. In itself, coumarin does not inhibit coagulation, but through fermentation it is changed to dicoumarin that does. In humans, the vitamin K factor inhibits this response.

Fresh sweet clover has low levels of free coumarin, but cis and trans-0-hydroxycinnamic acid glucosides are stored in vacuoles and when ruptured, an endogenous B-glycosidase specific to cis-glycoside hydrolyses the latter to coumarinic acid, and lactonises to coumarin.

This B-glycosidase remains efficient in dry material and during water extraction at room temperature.

If sweet clover tea is taken for any length of time for anti-coagulant activity, combine with alfalfa or nettles, which are rich in vitamin K.

Potential for toxicity in humans is quite low, assuming normal liver function. Coumarin is metabolized to 7-hydroxycoumarin, not 3-hydroxycoumarin, as in rats and dog studies.

Dicoumarol, or melitoxin, is only produced when fermentation takes place, due to fungal infection from *Aspergillus* or *Penicillium* species or spoilage.

Melilot contains constituents favorable for treating varicose veins, hemorrhoids, heavy leg syndrome, or thromophlebitis.

Sweet clover's action consists of decreasing the permeability of capillaries, while increasing venous, thoracic duct and lymphatic flow rates. It also stimulates portal circulation, which helps to clear congestion and toxicity in the liver.

Adolf Oerel and Eduard Bauer write, "due to its constituents, yellow sweet clover is excellent for treating varicose veins, cramp-like vascular pain in the arms and acute cramp in the lower leg."

A cup of sweet clover tea before bedtime will often stop excessive menstruation.

A number of studies have shown the action extends to the lymphatic ducts making it a useful treatment for lymphoedema, and swellings of the lymphatic glands.

It combines well with horse chestnut, linden flower, or hawthorn for phlebitis, thrombo-phlebitis and other varicosities.

It can be used both internally and externally as a poultice or fomentation for hot painful swelling from boils, injury, lymphatic swelling and breast lumps or mastitis.

In an open study, a melilot extract (20 mg containing 4 mg coumarin) was given to 25 women with lymphoedema, following breast cancer surgery, for 12 weeks. Marked reduction in swelling was noted after six weeks and at end of trial highly significant results were noted. Muraca et al, *Gazz Med Ital Arch Sci Med* 1999 158.

Another open study of 17 patients with same conditions showed benefit. Pastura et al, *Clin Terr* 1999 150.

Coumarins reduce high protein edema by increasing pumping of collecting lymphatics but also via macrophage stimulation.

In chronic lymphoedema, macrophages are dormant or less active and coumarins restore normal activity. They promote proteolysis and the fragments are re-absorbed directly back into the bloodstream. Casley-Smith et al, *Lymphology* 1988 21.

Overall, the action of sweet clover includes two special effects on the nervous system. One is systemic, inhibiting the sympathetic nervous system, making it useful and calming for insomnia in children and the elderly.

The other effect is relaxing and anti-spasmodic. For chronic bronchitis conditions it is similar in action to self heal. For this reason it is often in medicinal herbal cigarettes for bronchial asthma. This same effect works well for flatulent colic and other digestive spasms.

Drop doses of the tincture were given traditionally by country doctors, for seizures. The early Eclectic physicians recommended Melilotus for spasmodic pain associated with muscle weakness, and cold hands and fingers that are tender to the touch.

Polysaccharides from the plant show immune modulating, anti-anemic and adaptogenic properties. Pokdolzin et al, *Bull Exp Biol Med* 1996 121.

The seeds contain dicoumarol, active against broad-spectrum bacteria; as well as possessing anti-estrogenic and anti-phlogistic action. Dicoumarol is a potent anti-coagulant, and should be used with caution.

A 1993 study by Maucher et al, found clover coumarins inhibit prostate cancer growth. Various isocoumarins act as gastric protectives, due to an increase in prostaglandin production. Goel et al, *Ind J Exp Biol* 1997 35.

In a 1987 study by Marshall et al, 45 metastatic renal cell cancer patients were given 100 mg per day of clover coumarin and 300 mg cimetide 4 times daily. Results showed both to be safe and effective for treatment of the disease.

Thornes et al, *European Journal of Surgical Oncology* 1989 15:5 found coumarin stimulated macrophages and reduced recurrence of metastatic melanoma in a study on 27 patients.

In Russia, a standardized tablet is available containing 0.43-0.46 mg flavonoids and 0.109-0.110 mg coumarin.

Infused leaves can be used for eye inflammation, stomach pains, and headaches. Facial, ovarian and intercostal neuralgia; as well as sciatic pain responds.

Use both internally and externally in baths, or in the form of compresses and fomentations; especially if aggravated by cold. The flower heads are particularly anti-spasmodic.

Sitz baths give relief to tissue after childbirth, rectal, vaginal or uterine surgery, and interstitial cystitis, according to Michael Moore.

Sleep pillows contain yellow clover for driving away melancholy.

It's natural vanilla flavour and odor improve the taste of many herbal blends.

Several patents exist for anti-inflammatory skin ointments.

One study looked at 0.25% coumarin yellow sweet clover extract for reducing inflammation. They found it reduced the activation of circulating phagocytes and lowered citrulline production, working in a manner similar to, but milder than, hydrocortisone. Plesca-Manea et al, *Phyto Research* 2002 16:4.

Coumarin is used in cosmetics as a skin decongestant, astringent. Use an infusion for decongesting the eyelids and periocular zone.

Studies on water extracts of Yellow Sweet Clover leaf indicate activity against myco-bacteria. White Sweet Clover extracts from the flowers, leaves and roots by ether, acetone, alkaline or water show activity against mycobacterium as well as gram negative and gram positive bacteria.

White Sweet Clover extracts were found, in rat studies, to greatly reduce swelling, necrosis and induration of injured leg skin after a burn.

White Sweet Clover seeds have been studied in Russia, and found to contain low molecular weight anti-oxidants, with high peroxidase levels; especially when gathered during periods of high heat and low precipitation. The same study, by Stognii in Russia, found seeds from Yarrow (*A. millefolium*) contained high SOD levels.

Interesting research was conducted by Bondarenko in Russia in 1973. Sweet Clover leaves were kept at 2-4°C in darkness and analyzed for constituents. While many constituents decreased or remained the same, organic and melilotic acids increased.

The seeds contain canavanin, and like alfalfa, ingestion may cause exaggeration of symptoms in those affected by the auto-immune disease lupus. See Alfalfa in Musculo-skeletal system.

HOMEOPATHY

Yellow and white melilotus is specific for congestion and hemorrhage of the blood system. Congestive and nervous headaches may be present. Epilepsy created by blow to the head is another indication for its usage. In tincture or 1X potency, it is specific for those headaches and optic neuralgia that drive patients so wild they bang their heads into the wall or floor.

There may be vomiting, as well as cold hands and feet with the headache. The face may be flushed and red, with scanty menses and ovarian neuralgia and pain. Hypertension, caused by kidney weakness, is reduced.

Emotionally, melilotus is for those who anger easily, are impatient, dissatisfied-satisfied and have an intellectual slowness. Want to run away, kill himself, kill those who approach. Think there is a devil in stomach, compulsive disorders, fear of poverty, danger and police, constant prayer, insanity from grief.

All symptoms of the melilotus individual are made worse on rainy, changeable days, about 4 PM and approaching storm.

DOSE-tincture and lower potencies. The mother tincture is prepared from the fresh leaves and flowers. Proving by Bowen with tincture and 1C as well as effects of chewing plant and smelling flowers. Both white and yellow were used in 1866 study.

Melilotus alba is for an inability to fix the mind, they speak incoherently, impatient, fault-finding, suspicious, fear of poverty, stricken with panic, dreams full of contention and bickering. Insomnia or unable to sleep after 3 am, anorexia in morning, very hungry by 10 am.

Tension and wave-like motion in brain, intense frontal headaches, and excessive dryness of nose.

DOSE- lower potencies to 30C. Proving by Allen with two females and four males at 30c in 1886.

ESSENTIAL OIL

CONSTITUENTS- coumarins- melilotic acid and orthocoumaric acid.

A concrete is usually made from the dried flowers by solvent extraction. It is viscous dark green with a "new-mown hay" scent. This oleoresin is used in high-class perfume and in flavouring tobacco where coumarin is not banned.

It is used as an absolute or oleoresin in perfumes for forest and field like blends, and to help round off synthetic preparations. It blends well with fir needle absolute, and oakmoss.

The essential oil is steam distilled from the yellow, flowering tops, yielding 0.0133%. It is prized for it's calming and relaxing effect. It contains thirty-five compounds with the major one coumarin at 35.3% followed by (Z)-3-hexen-1-ol at 26%.

Medicinally, it is used for its urinary diuretic and antiseptic action. For circulatory problems involving fat deposits in the arteries and veins, it is beneficial; and for thrombosis, it may be added to external massage blends.

A sun infused oil can be made with fresh flowers and used for sore muscles. When mixed with a little beeswax to firm it up, it can be used successfully in treating chronic eczema.

A Sweet Clover ointment, such as *Le Thalasso Bain Leg Health Gel* by Goemar, may be used to increase lymphatic flow in lymphoedema by daily application to affected tissue.

HYDROSOL

CONSTITUENTS- *M. officinalis*- eucalyptol 26%, p-menthone 22%, camphor 16%, dimethyl sulphide 9%, cis-Thujone 10%, menthol 3.4% and minor amounts of bornyl acetate, linalool, and isomenthone, endo borneol, trans thujone, and both terpenin-4-ol and alpha terpineol.

Grieve mentions that the water distilled from Sweet Clover flower improves the flavour of other ingredients in a combination.

Viaud mentions that the traditional uses of the distilled water as an antispasmodic, anticoagulant, and used for phlebitis, embolism and blocked circulation is confirmed.

Brunschwig recommended the water for those who anger easily and for all those that would govern themselves by wisdom.

The head often washed with the distilled water of the herb and flowers...is effectual for those that have suddenly lost their senses, as also to strengthen the memory, comfort the head and brain, and to preserve them from pains and apoplexy. **CULPEPPER**

From firsthand experience, people long ago attributed to the distilled water of melilot in particular such virtues as strengthening the head and memory and purifying the kidneys and bladder of sand and gravel, when three loths of it were drunk in the evening before going to bed. **SAUER**

SEED OIL

The seed oil yields 8.3%, and is composed of palmitic acid (4.6%), stearic acid (3.3%), oleic acid (12.7%), linoleic (63.2%), linolenic (14.7%), and arachidic acid (1.3%).

FLOWER ESSENCES

Sweet clover flower essence is for those who have suffered loss of memory, or need emotional comfort from the fear and pain of stroke. They are unable to think clearly or concentrate. They want to run away and hide; or may suffer delusions and paranoia. **PRAIRIE DEVA**

Yellow sweet flower is good for nervousness, stress and tension/ aggression. Sunny, carefree, helps one to feel like "Polyanna" and see the glass half full instead of half empty. Helps you to look for the silver lining in every cloud, and if you can't find one, it's only temporary anyway. **RAVENWORKS**

SPIRITUAL PROPERTIES

The major quality lacking among mankind is the ability to "understand with the heart". This would allow many souls to accept that all things have meaning and that the events through which they pass are intended to broaden and render more spiritual the outlook they bring to reality. The tiny flowers, when mashed into gruel and eaten cold, promote an opening of this wellspring of heart-centered wisdom, and quicken the grasp of truth which is known by the heart alone. **HILARION**

Like her scent, sweet clover has a countenance that is light and full of grace-never heavy and earthy. She is so delicately proportioned that one could almost overlook her, or rather look through her. She would almost seem to take off and float if her deep growing taproot did not anchor her securely on Earth.

Sweet Clover, of old, was considered a gentle plant of feminine beauty and purity. In ancient Greece she was dedicated to the nine beautiful daughters of Jupiter and Mnemosyne, the graceful muses and goddesses of song and poetry and the arts and sciences.

We know the ancient Germans assigned her to Ostara (Eostre), the goddess of light, fertility and spring. They celebrated her feast day in April, lighting Easter bonfires to symbolize the "rising up of the light" following winter's darkness. The women braided wreaths from flowering yellow sweet clover to throw on the flames.

Of course, the Blessed Mary eventually supplanted the old icon. Today, while few people still recognize the old connection between human, animal, and plant kingdoms, a growing number understand the values that moved women herbalists of the past. **FISCHER-RIZZI**

PERSONALITY TRAITS

[Sweet clover] are acting as if they are hiding, and talk in whispers so as not to be noticed or discovered. They are living out the story of Anne Frank hiding in the attic in real life. Inside are feelings of being watched, looked at, in great danger and being pursued by enemies.

PETER CHAPPELL

Dr. Bowen says he in the habit of prescribing it [Melilotus] for all cases of insanity, to reduce the hyperaemic condition of the brain, thinking he would use the indicated remedy as soon as the acute congestion was removed, but found that Melilotus cured the entire train of mental symptoms and restored the patient to health...I call the attention of members to these mental symptoms of Melilotus because there are few remedies that may be more useful in the treatment of insanity and mental affections. **ALLEN**

RECIPES

TINCTURE- 1-50 drops of a 1:5 recently dried leaf and flower tincture at 40% alcohol. Since coumarin quickly breaks down to umbelliferone in human metabolism, the best results occur from either frequent use (say 6-8 times daily) or from slow release preparations.

Lymphselect® is a 20% coumarin product with recommended dose of 20-50 mg daily.

Herb has a half-life of 2.5 days in body.

POWDER- Up to 60 grains.

INFUSION- Pour eight ounces of boiling water over 1-2 tsps of dried plant. Strain after 15-20 minutes. Drink 2-3 cups daily. You can also apply as a cold compress to broken capillaries on the face, and to firm the tissue.

SWEET CLOVER LIQUEUR- Take one half cup of sweet clover leaves and flowers dried; one half cup of dried linden or basswood leaves (fresh or dried), one half cup of dried rose leaves, and one vanilla bean in a mason jar.

Dissolve four tablespoons of honey in a small amount of any fruit liqueur and pour over the herbs. Fill with the rest of 500 ml of liqueur and steep covered for three weeks. Strain and let stand for two more months before serving.

CAUTION- Do not use sweet clover if using prescription warfarin or other blood thinners, salicylates, or if you suffer from anemia. Do not use before giving birth or surgery for the same reason. Avoid the seeds in cases of lupus.

Standardized extracts are usually 17.9% coumarin content.
Liver enzymes should be monitored if used long term, as well as prothrombin time.

Michael Moore suggests there are no contraindications. "Even though I have warned against excessive use of such a coumarin-containing herb, following accepted semi-scientific Conventional Wisdom, I was wrong, and so is the CW."

Warfarin interferes with the production of prothrombin in the liver when given in repeated small doses. The capillaries are also damaged. The stresses of normal life are then sufficient to produce fatal hemorrhage following very slight trauma to capillaries or small blood vessels.

ABOUT THE AUTHOR

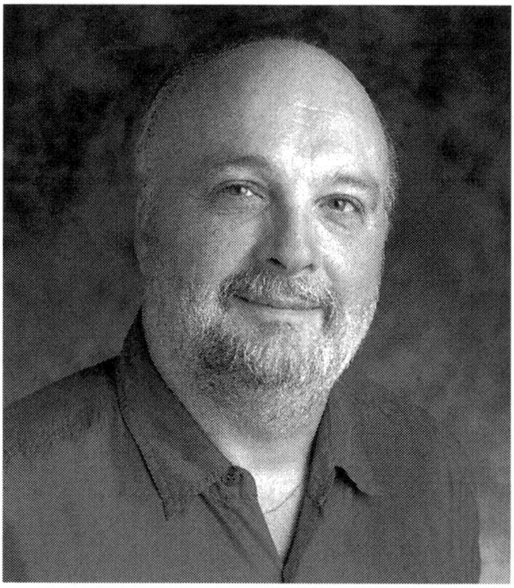

Robert Dale Rogers has been an herbalist for over forty years. He has a Bachelor of Science from the University of Alberta, where he is an assistant clinical professor in Family Medicine. He teaches plant medicine, including herbology and flower essences at Grant MacEwan University, as well as Earth Spirit Medicine at the Northern Star College of Mystical Studies in Edmonton, Alberta, Canada.

Robert is past chair of the Alberta Natural Health Agricultural Network and Community Health Council of Capital Health. He is a Fellow of the International College of Nutrition, chair of the medicinal mushroom committee of the North American Mycological Association and on the editorial board of the International Journal of Medicinal Mushrooms, and Discovery Phytomedicine.

Robert co-hosts The Alberta Herb Gathering held every second year (www.albertaherbgathering.com)

He lives on Millcreek Ravine in Edmonton with his beautiful and talented wife, Laurie Szott-Rogers and out of control cat Ceres.

You can email him at scents@telusplanet.net
or visit
www.selfhealdistributing.com

BIBLIOGRAPHY

Abbe, Elfriede, The Fern Herbal, Cornell University Press, Ithaca, 1981
Acorn, J. Bugs of Alberta, Lone Pine Publishing, Edmonton, AB, 2000.
Adams, J. Les Plantes Medicinales. Bulletin 23, Agriculture Canada. 1916
Adams, Jean. Insect Potpourri, Adventures in Entomology. Sandhill Crane Press, FL. 1992
Aggarwal, Bharat. Healing Spices. Sterling Pub. New York 2011.
Albert-Puleo, Michael. Economic Botany, 32, Jan-Mar, 1978.
Allaby, Michael. Temperate Forests. Facts on File. New York. 1999.
Allen, D & Hatfield, G. Medicinal Plants in Folk Tradition. Timber Press, Portland. 2004
Allen,E, Morrison,D, &Wallis,G. Common Tree Diseases of B.C. Canada Forest Service, '96
Allende, Isabel. Aphrodite- A Memoir of the Senses. Harper Flamingo. New York. 1998.
Alstat, Ed. Electic Dispensatory of Botanical Therapeutics. Ecl Med. Oregon. 1989.
Anderson, Anne, Some Native Herbal Remedies, Pub 8A, Devonian Botanical Gardens 1980
_____ Plants in Cree. Duval House Pub. Edmonton AB 2000.
Anderson, C.&Tischer,T. Poinsettias, the December Flower, Waters Edge Press, CA, 1997
Andoh, Anthony. The Science & Romance of Selected Herbs used in Medicine and Religious Ceremony. North Scale Institute. San Francisco. 1986.
Andre, Alestine & Fehr, Alan. Gwich'in Ethnobotany. Gwich'in Social and Cultural Institute, Box 46, Tsiigehtchie, NWT, X0E 0B0, fax 1867-953-3820.
Andrews, Tamra. Nectar and Ambrosia. ABC-CLIO Box 1911 Santa Barbara CA. 2000.
Andrews, Ted. Animal Speak- The Spiritual and Magical Powers, Llewellyn. Minn. 1996.
_____ Animal Wise, DragonHawk, Jackson, TN, 1999.
Antol, Marie. The Incredible Secrets of Mustard. Avery Pub. New York. 1999.
Aronson J K Ed. Meyler's Side Effects of Herbal Medicines. Elsevier Amsterdam. 2009.
Arrowsmith, Nancy. Essential Herbal Wisdom. Llewellyn Pub. Woodbury, Minn. 2009.
Arsdall, Anne Van. Medieval Herbal Remedies. Routledge, New York. 2002.
Arvigo & Balick, Rainforest Remedies, Lotus Press, Twin Lakes, WI. 1993
Arvigo & Epstein. Rainforest Home Remedies, Harper SanFrancisco, 2001.
Assiniwi, Bernard. La Medecine des Indiens d'Amerique, Guerin Literature, 1988
Atal C.K. & Kapur B. Cultivation and Utilization of Medicinal Plants, Jammu-Tawi, 1982
Attenborough, David. The Private Life of Plants. Princeton U Press. Princeton NJ 1995.
Ausubel, K. Seeds of Change The Living Treasure. HarperSanFrancisco, 1994.
Aversano, Laura. The Divine Nature of Plants. Swan•Raven & Co. Columbus, NC, 2002.
Ayensu, Edward,S. Medicinal Plants of the West Indies, Reference Publications, 1981
Baïracli Levy, Juliette Herbal Handbook for Farm and Stable, Faber&Faber, London, 1952
Baker, Phil. The Dedalus Book of Absinthe. Dedalus 2001.
Barl, Branka et al, Saskatchewan Herb Database, U. of Sask. Saskatoon, 1996.
Barlow, Max. From the Shepherd's Purse. 1990
Barnes J, Anderson L, &Phillipson J. Herbal Medicines, A guide for healthcare professionals. Pharmaceutical Press, London, 2002.
Barnett, Robert A. Tonics, Harper Collins, New York, N.Y. 1997
Bartram, Thomas. Bartram's Encyl. of Herbal Medicine, Robinson Pub. London, 1998.
Bascom, Angella. Incorporating Herbal Medicine into Clinical Practice. F. Davis Co. 2002
Beals, Katherine, M. Flower Lore and Legend, Henry Holt, 1917
Beers, Susan-Jane. Jamu The ancient Indonesian Art of Herbal Healing, Periplus, 2001.
Belcourt, Christi. Medicines to Help Us. Gabriel Dumont Instit. Saskatoon, SK 2007.
Béliveau, R & Gingras,D. Foods That Fight Cancer. McClelland & Stewart Toronto. 2006.
Belsinger S & Dille C. Cooking with Herbs. CBI- Van Nostrand Reinhold, N.Y. 1984.

Benjamin, D.R. Mushrooms: Poisons and Panaceas. WH Freeman, San Francisco, 1995.
Bennet, Doug & Tiner, Tim. Up North. Reed Books Canada. Markham, Ont. 1993.
_____ Up North Again. McClelland and Stewart. Toronto, 1997.
Bennet, J & Rowley S. Uqalurait An Oral History of Nunavut. McGill Queens, Mont. 2004
Benyus, Janine. Biomimicry Innovation Inspired by Nature. William Morrow. 1997.
Berenbaum,May R. Buzzwords, A Scientists Muses on Sex, Bugs and Rock N Roll, Joseph Henry Press, Washington, D.C. 2000.
_____ Bugs in the System. Helix Books, Addison-Wesley Pub. 1995.
Beresford-Kroeger, Diana. The Global Forest. Viking Penguin. 2010.
_____ Arboretum Borealis. U Michigan Press. 2010.
Berliocchi,Luigi. The Orchid in Lore and Legend. Timber Press, Portland Oregon, 2000.
Berlund B & Bolsby C. The Edible Wild Pagurian Press, Toronto, Ont. 1971.
Berkowsky, Bruce. Mount Julius Flower Remedies. Mt. Vernon Washington, 1986
Bermejo, J & Leon,J. Neglected Crops-1492 ... FAO Series 26, United Nations, Rome, 1994.
Bernhardt, P. The Rose's Kiss, A Natural History of Flowers . Island Press, Covelo CA 1999
Bianchi, Ivo. Geriatrics and Homotoxicology. Aurelia-Verlag GmbH, Baden Baden, 1994.
Bianchini, F. The Complete Book of Health Plants. Crescent Books, New York, 1975.
Biship, Carol. The Book of Home Remedies &Herbal Cures, Jonathan-James, Toronto, 1979.
Bisset, Norman G. Herbal Drugs and Phytopharmaceuticals. 2nd Ed. CRC Press, 2001.
Blackburn, Thomas. December's Child: A Book of Chumash Oral Narratives , U of California Press, Berkeley, 1975.
Blanchan, Neltje. Nature's Garden. Doubleday, Page&Co. New York, 1900.
Bland, John. Forests of Liliput. Prentice Hall, Englewood Cliffs, New Jersey, 1971.
Bliss, Anne. Rocky Mountain Dye Plants. Juniper House, Boulder, Colorado, 1976
Blouin, Glen. Weeds of the Woods. Goose Lane, Fredericton, New Brunswick 1992.
_____ An Eclectic Guide to Trees, east of the Rockies. Boston Mills, 2001.
Boas, F. Ethnology of the Kwakiutl. Bureau of Am. Ethnology, 35th annual report, 1921.
Boericke, Wm. Materia Medica with Repetory. B. Jain Publishers. 1976
Boik, John. Natural Compunds in Cancer Therapy. Oregon Med Press, Princeton,Minn 2001
Boland, Bridget. Gardener's Magic &Other Old Wives' Lore. The Bodley Head, London, 77.
Bolton, Brett L. The Secret Powers of Plants. Berkley Pub Co. New York. 1974.
Bolton, J.L. Alfalfa, Botany, Cultivation &Utilization. Interscience Pub, New York, 1962.
Bone, Kerry. A Clinical Guide to Blending Liquid Herbs. Churchill Livingstone. 2003
Borrel, Marie. Healing Plants. Cassell & Co. Wellington House, London. 2001.
Bouchardon, Patrice. The Healing Energies of Trees. Journey Editions, Boston, 1999.
Bossenmaier, Eugene. Mushrooms of the Boreal Forest. U. of Saskatchewan Press, 1997
Boulos, Loutfy. Medicinal Plants of North Africa, Reference Pub. Algonac, Mich. 1983
Bowles, E. Joy. The Chemistry of Aromatherapeutic Oils. Allen & Unwin, Crow's Nest, Australia, 2003.
Bowman, Daria. Hydrangeas. Friedman/Fairfax Pub. New York. 1999.
Bradley, Peter. British Herbal Compendium Vol 2 Brit Herb Med Assoc. Bournemouth 2006.
Brahmachari, Goutam Ed. Natural Products, Alpha Sci Int Ltd. Oxford UK 2009.
Brandeis, Gayle. Fruitflesh. Harper Collins, San Francisco. 2002.
Brennan, M. Complete Holistic Care & Healing for Horses. Trafalgar Sq. Pub. VT. 2001.
Bringhurst, Robert. A Story as Sharp as a Knife. Douglas&McIntyre Vancouver, 1999.
Brinker, Francis N.D. Herb Contraindications and Drug Interactions .Third Edition Eclectic Medical Publications, Sandy, Oregon, 2001
_____ The Toxicology of Botanical Medicines, revised 2nd. Eclectic Med, Oregon, 1996.
_____ Eclectic Dispensatory of Botanical Therapeutics, Vol 2, Ecl. Med . Oregon, 1995.
Brodo, Irwin & Sharnoff. Lichens of North America. Yale University Press, 2001.

Brown, Deni. Enclyclopedia of Herbs and Their Uses. Reader's Digest Press, Que. 1995.
Bruneton, J Pharmacognosy, Phtyochemistry, Medicinal Plants, Lavoisier Pub. Paris, 1995
_____ Toxic Plants Dangerous to Humans and Animals. Editions TEC&Doc, Paris, '99.
Brunschwig, Hieronymus. Book of Distillation. Johnson Reprint Co No. 79. New York, 1971.
Bubar, Carol et al. Weeds of the Prairies. Alberta Agriculture Pub. Edmonton, 2000.
Buchanan, Carol. Brothers Crow, Sister Corn. Ten Speed Press, Berkeley, 1997.
Buckle, Jane. Clinical Aromatherapy. 2nd ed. Churchill Livingstone, Toronto, 2003.
Buhner, Stephen H. Sacred and Herbal Healing Beers, Siris Books, Boulder, Co, 1998
_____ Sacred Plant Medicine. Robert Rinehart, Boulder, Co. 1996.
_____ Herbal Antibiotics. Storey Books, Vermont, 1999.
_____ The Lost Language of Plants. Chelsea Green Pub. White River, Vt. 2002
_____ Secret Teachings of Plants. Bear & Co. Rochester, Vt. 2004.
_____ The Natural Testosterone Plan. Healing Arts Press, Rochester VT. 2007
Burbridge, Joan. Wildflowers of the Southern Interior of B.C. U. of B.C. Press, 1989.
Burger, W. Flowers- How they changed the world. Prometheus Books. Amherst NY 2006.
Burgess, Isla. Weeds Heal. Viriditas Pub Group. Cambridge NZ 1998.
Burlando, Bruno et al, Herbal Principles in Cosmetics. CRC Press Boca Raton 2010.
Caius, Rev. Fr. Jean F., The Medicinal and Poisonous Plants of India, Scientific Pub, 1986.
Cameron, Elizabeth. A Floral ABC. John Wiley and Sons. Toronto. 1980.
Carpenter D. Snr Pub. Nursing Herbal Medicine Handbook, Springhouse Corp. 2001.
Carpinella, Maria et al. Novel Therapeutic Agents from Plants. Sci Pub. Enfield NJ 2009.
Carr, Emily. Wild Flowers. Royal BC Museum, Victoria, B.C, 2006
Carroll, Roisin. The Crane Bag Celtic Tree Ogam Oils , Feasibility Pub. Dublin
Carter, Bernard F. The Floral Birthday Book. Bloomsbury Books, London. 1990.
Casselman, Bill. Canadian Garden Words. Little, Brown & Co. Toronto, 1997.
Castleman, Michael. The Healing Herbs. Bantam Books. 1995.
Castro, Miranda. The Complete Homeopathy Handbook. MacMillan, 1990
Catty, Suzanne. Hydrosols the next Aromatherapy, Healing Arts Press, Vermont, 2001.
Cavers, Paul ed, The Biology of Canadian Weeds 62-83,Ag Institute of Canada, Ottawa, 1995
_____ 84-102 Ag Inst. of Canada, Ottawa, 2000.
_____ 103-129 Ag Inst. of Canada, Ottawa 2005
Ceres. Herbal Teas for Health and Healing. Healing Arts Press, Rochester, Vermont, 1984.
Chan, K, and Cheung L. Interactions between Chincese Herbal Medicinal Products and Orthodox Drugs. Harwood Academic Publishers, Canada, 2000.
Chandler, F. Herbs-Everyday Reference for Health Professionals, Can. Pharm Assoc. 2000
Chang & But. Pharmacology &Applications of Chinese Materia Medica, World Scientific, 86
Chang Chao-liang et al, Vegetables as Medicine, Pelanduk Pub, Malaysia, 1999.
Chappell, P. Emotional Healing with Homeopathy. North Atlantic Books. Berkeley, 2003.
Chase, Pamela & Pawlik, J. Newcastle Trees for Healing , Newcastle Pub. Van Nuys,1991
Chatroux, Sylvia. Botanica Poetica. Poetica Press 2004 1-877-POETICA.
_____ Materica Poetica. Poetica Press 1998.
Chen, John K & Chen, Tina T. Chinese Medical Herbology & Pharmacology. Art of Medicine Press, City of Industry, CA 2004.
Chevalllier, Andrew. The Encyclopedia of Medicinal Plants. Reader's Digest, 1996.
Chishti, Hakim. The Traditional Healer, Healing Arts Press, Vermont,1988.
Clark, Ella E. Indian Legends of Canada. McClelland & Stewart. Toronto, 1960.
Coats, Peter. Flowers in History. Weidenfeld and Nicolson, London. 1970.
Coffey, Timothy.The History and Folklore of North American Wildflowers, Houghton-Mifflin, 1993.
Cohen, Kenneth. Honoring the Medicine. Random House, Toronto. 2003.

Conrad, Chris, Hemp for Health, Healing Arts Press, Rochester, Vermont, 1997.
Cook, Wm.H. The Physio-Medical Dispensatory. 1869. Reprinted by Eclectic Medical Publications, Portland, Oregon, 1985.
_____ A compendium of the new Materia medica together with additional descriptions of some old remedies. Wm. Cook Publisher, Chicago, 1896.
Cooper, J.C. Dictionary of Symbolic & Mythological Animals, Thorsons, London, 1992.
Cormack, R.G.H. Wild Flowers of Alberta. Hurtig Publishers, 1977
Coupland, Francois. The Encyclopedia of Edible Plants of N. America. Keats Pub. 1998.
Cousin, Pierre J. Eat Well, Be Well. Thorsons, London. 2001.
Cowan, Eliot. Plant Spirit Medicine. Swan Raven & Co. Box 726 Newberg, Oregon, 1995.
Cowan, Thomas. The Fourfold Path to Healing. New Trends Pub. Washington DC 2007.
Crane, Eva. Honey- A Comprhensive Survey , Heinemann Pub. London 1975.
Craydon D. & Bellows W. Floral Acupuncture. The Crossing Press Berkeley CA 2005.
Creekmore, H. Daffodils are Dangerous. Walker and Co. New York. 1966.
Crow, Tis Mal. Native Plants, Native Healing. Native Voices Book Pub. Box 99 Summertown, Tennessee, 2001 1-888-260-8458.
Crowell, Robert L. The Lore & Legends of Flowers. Thomas Crowell, New York, 1982.
Crowfoot & Baldensperger. From Cedar to Hyssop. Sheldon Press, London, 1932.
Cruden, Loren. Medicine Grove. Destiny Books. Inner Traditions Vermont. 1997.
Cummings, S. and Ullman, Dana. Everyone's Guide to Homeopathic Medicines, St. Martins
Cupp, Melanie. Toxicology and Clinical Pharmacology of Herbal Products. Humana P. 1999
Curtin, LSM. Healing Herbs of the Upper Rio Grande. SouthWest Museum, Los Angeles 1965
Cutler & Cutler Eds. Biologically Active Natural Products: Agrochemicals, CRC Press 1999.
Dai Yin-fang&Liu Cheng-jun. Fruit As Medicine. Rams Skull Press, Kuranda, Aust. 1987
Dalton, David. Stars of the Meadow. Lindisfarne Books. Great Barrington, Mass. 2006.
D'Amelio Sr. Frank. Botanicals A Phytocosmetic Desk Reference CRC Press, Boca Raton, 99
Darby,Wm et al. Food: The Gift of Osiris, Vol 1. Academic Press, San Francisco, 1977
Darwin, Tess. The Scots Herbal, the Plant Lore of Scotland. Birlinn Ltd, Edinburgh 2008
Davidow, Joie. Infusions of Healing, A Treasury of Mexican-American Herbal Remedies, Fireside Books, New York, 1999.
Davis,W. El Gringo, New Mexico and Her People. Harpers, New York, 1857.
Demargaux, N. Phytotherapy. Herbal Health Publishers Ltd. 1989
De Bairacli Levy, Juliette. Herbal Handbook for Farm and Stable, Faber and Faber 1952
Deer Lame, J & Erdoes, R. Lame Deer Seeker of Visions. Washington Sq Press, 1976.
Deer, Thea Summer. Wisdom of the Plant Devas. Bear&Company Vermont 2011.
De Smet et al. Adverse Effects of Herbal Drugs. Springer-Verlag, Berlin. 1997.
Der Marderosian, Ara & Liberti L. Natural Product Medicine, George Stickley Co, Philadel.
Diederichsen, Axel. Coriander. Int. Plant Genetic Resources Institute. Rome, Italy. 1996.
DeRios, Marlene D. Hallucinogens: Cross Cultural Perspectives. U. New Mexico Press, 1984
DeSmet, P. et al. Adverse Effects of Herbal Drugs. vol 2 Springer-Verlag
Devi, Lila. The Essential Flower Essence Handbook. Crystal Clarity Pub. Nevada City 2007.
Dewey, Laurel. Plant Power- revised. Safe Goods/New Century Pub, Markham Ont, 2001.
Dewick, Paul M. Medicinal Natural Products.3rd Ed John Wiley and Sons, West Sussex, 2009.
Dixon, Bernard.Power Unseen, How Microbes Rule the World. W.H. Freeman, Oxford, 1994
Dow, Elaine. Simples and Worts. Historical Presentations, Topsfield, MA. 1982.
Duke, James. Handbook of Medicinal Herbs. CRC Press, Boca Raton, Florida, 1985
_____ Handbook of Edible Weeds. CRC Press. 1992
_____ The Green Pharmacy, Rodale Press, Emmaus, Pennsylvania, 1997.
_____ The Green Pharmacy Herbal Handbook, Rodale Press, 2000.

_____ Anti-aging Prescriptions. Rodale Press. 2001.
Dumas, Anne. Book of Plants and Symbols. English Ed. Octopus Pub. London 2004.
Dymock,Wm. Pharmacographia Indica, Vol 2, Kegan Paul, Trench, Trubner and Co. 1891
Earle, Liz. Vital Oils, Ebury Press, London, 1991.
Eason, Cassandra. Fabulous Creatures, Mythical Monsters... Greenwood Press, CT. 2008.
Eastman, John. The Book of Swamp and Bog... Stackpole Books, Mechanicsburg, Penn, 1995
Ebadi, M. Pharmacodynamic Basis of Herbal Medicine, CRC Press, Boca Raton. 2002.
Eckey, E.W. Vegetable Fats and Oils, Rheingold Publishing Co, New York, 1954.
Eclare, Melanie. Flower Spirit Cards. Quadrille Publishing, London, England, 2004.
Edwards, Lawrence. The Vortex of Life. Floris Books. Edinburgh 2nd Ed. 2006.
Eisner T et al. Secret Weapons. Belknap Press, Harvard U Press. Cambridge & London 2005.
Ellingwood F. American Materia Medica, Eclectic Med. Pub. Portand, Oregon, reprint, 1983
Elliot, Douglas B. Roots . Chatham Press, Old Greenwich Conneticut.
Ellis, Hattie. Sweetness & Light. Hodder and Stoughton, London, 2004.
Erdoes & Ortiz. American Indian Myths and Legends, Pantethon Books, New York, 1984.
Erichsen-Brown,Charlotte. Use of Plants for the Past 500 Years, Breezy Creeks Press, 1979
_____ Medicinal and Other Uses of North American Plants, General Pub, 1979.
Erickson, David, Wai Kit Nip Food uses of whole oil and protein seeds, Amer. Oil Chemists Society, 1989.
Eskin, N. A. Michael, Tamir, S. Dictionary of Nutraceuticals and Functional Foods. CRC Press, 2006.
Etkin, Nina. Edible Medicines, An Ethnopharmacology of Food. U Arizona Press. 2006.
Evans, W.C. Trease and Evans' Pharmacognosy. WB Saunders Co. Toronto, 2000.
Fang Jing Pei, Dr. Natural Remedies from the Chinese Cupboard. Weatherhill, 1998.
Farmer-Knowles,Helen. The Healing Garden. Sterling Publishing, New York, 1998.
Fielder, Mildred. Plant Medicne and Folklore, Winchester Press, New York, 1975.
Felter, Harvery and Lloyd, John. King's American Dispensatory . 1898.
Reprinted by Eclectic Medical Publications, Portland Oregon, 1983.
Ferguson, Gary. Spirits of the Wild. Clarkson Potter/Random New York, 1996.
Fernie, W.T. Dr. Old Fashioned Herbal Remedies. Coles Pub. Toronto, 1980. Reprint.
Fingerman M. et al editors. Bioremediation of Aquatic and Terresrial Ecosytems. Sci Pub. Enfield NH 2005.
Fischer-Rizzi, S. Complete Aromatherapy Handbook, Sterling Pub. New York. 1990.
_____ The Complete Incense Book, Sterling Pub. New York. 1998.
_____ Medicine of the Earth, Rudra Press, Portland, Oregon, 1996
Florey, H.W. et al. Antibiotics vol 1. Oxford University Press. London 1949.
Ford, Gillian. Plant Names Explained. Friends of the Devonian Botanic Garden, #16, 1984
Foster, Steven. Herbal Renaissance, Gibbs Smith Pub. Salt Lake City
_____ & Yue Chongxi. Herbal Emissaries, Healing Arts Press, Vermont, 1992
_____ & Johnson R. Desk Reference to Nature's Medicine. Nat Geographic. Washington, D.C.
Fox, H. M. Gardening with Herbs. Macmillan Pub. New York 1933.
Freeman, D. & Mongeau D. Nettles and More...Vol One. Self published 2nd printing 2009.
Freeman, Lyn. Mosby's Complementary & Alternative Medicine.3rd Ed. Mosby Elsevier 2009
Friedman, Sara Ann, Celebrating the Wild Mushroom, Dodd, Mead & Co. New York, 1986
Friend, Tim. The Third Domain: the Untold Story of Archaea. Joseph Henry Press. 2007.
Fugh-Berman, Adriane. The 5-minute Herb &Dietary Supplement Consult. Lippincott Williams &Wilkins, Philadelphia 2003.
Gaertner, Erika. Reap without Sowing. General Store Publishing, Burnstown, Ont. 1995
Galun, Margalith. Handbook of Lichenology, CRC Press, 1988

Garran, Thomas. Western herbs according to Traditional Chinese Medicine. Healing Arts Press. 2008.
Garrett, J.T. The Cherokee Herbal. Bear&Company, Rochester, Vermont. 2003.
Genders, Roy. Floral Scents of the World . St. Martin's Press, London, 1977
Geuter, Herbs in Nutrition. Bio-Dynamic Agricultural Assoc. London. 1978.
Gildemeister, E. The Volatile Oils. John Wiley and Sons, New York. 1916
Gifford, Jane. The Wisdom of Trees. Sterling Pub. New York 2000.
Gill S. & Sullivan I. Dictionary of Native American Mythology. Oxford U Press 1992.
Gilmore, M.R. Uses of Plants by Indians of the Missouri river region. 33rd Annual Report Bureau American Ethnology, 1911-12, Washington D.C. 1919.
Gladstar R & Hirsch P. Planting the Future. Healing Arts Press, Rochester, Vt. 2000.
Gladstar, Rosemary. Family Herbal. Storey Books, North Adams, Mass. 2001.
Glasby, J.S. Dictionary of Plants Containing Secondary Metabolites, Taylor & Francis, London 1991.
Godfrey, A & Saunders P. Principles and Practices of Naturopathic Botanical Medicine, Vol 1, CCNM Press Toronto ON 2010.
Goodrick-Clarke, Clare. Alchemical Medicine for the 21st Century. Healing Arts Press. 2010.
Gordon, David G. The Compleat Cockroach. Ten Speed Press, Berkeley, CA. 1996.
Gordon, Lesley. The Mystery and Magic of Trees & Flowers. Grange Books. London 1993.
Gottesfeld, Leslie M. Johnson. Plants, Land and People, A Study of Wet'suwet'en Ethnobotany.U of A, 1993.
Grae, Ida. Nature's Colors, Dyes From Plants. Macmillan Pub. New York, 1974.
Graham, Frances K. Plant lore of an Alaskan Island. Alaska Northwest Pub. 1985
Grange, Michael etal, Handbook of Plants with Pest Control Properties, J. Wiley& Son 1988
Gray, Bev. The Boreal Herbal. Wild Food & Medicine Plants of the North. Aroma Borealis Press 2011
Green, James. The Male Herbal . Crossing Press, Freedom, California, 1991.
_____ The Herbal Medicine-Maker's Handbook. Crossing Press, Freedom CA 2000
Green, Jonathan. Consuming Passions. Sphere Books, London, 1985.
Grey Wolf. Earth Signs, Raincoast Books, Vancouver, B.C. 1998.
Grieve, M. A Modern Herbal. Jonathan Cape. 1931
Griffiths, Deirdre. Elk Island National Park. U. of Alberta Press, 1979.
Grigson, Geoffrey. A Herbal of All Sorts. Phoenix House, London
Grimaud, Baptiste,Paul. TAROT DES FLEURS, France Cartes, France 1989
Grimshaw, John. The Gardener's Atlas. Firefly Books, Willowdale, Ont. 2002.
Grohmann,Gerbert. The Plant Vol 2, Bio-Dynamic Farming & Gardening Assoc. 1989.
Gruenwald et al, Ed. PDR for Herbal Medicines. 4th Ed. Thomson Pub. 2007.
Guillet, Alma. Make Friends of Trees and Shrubs. Doubleday & Co. New York, 1962.
Gumbel, Dietrich. Principles of Holistic Skin Therapy with Herb Essences. Haug Pub. Heidelberg 1986.
Gurudas. The Spiritual Properties of Herbs , Cassandra Press, 1988
_____ Flower Essences and Vibrational Healing, Cassandra Press, 1983
Hageneder, Fred. The Spirit of Trees. Continuum. NY and London. 2005.
Hale, Mason. The Biology of Lichens. Edward Arnold Pub. London, 1967.
Hall, Dorothy. Creating Your Herbal Profile , Keats, 1988
Hallworth, B & Chinnappa CC. Plants of the Kananaskis Country U of A Press 1997.
Hanchuk, Rena. The Word and Wax. Can Inst of Ukrainian Studies Press, Edmonton, 1999.
Hanson, J, & Morrison D. Of Kinkajous, Capybaras, Horned Beetles...Harper Collins, NY '91
Harbourne & Baxter. The Handbook of Natural Flavonoids Vol 1&2. John Wiley & Sons, 1999
_____ Phytochemical Dictionary. Taylor & Francis 1993.

Harrington, Geri. Growing Your Own Chinese Vegetables, MacMillan, N.Y. 1978.
Harrington, H.D. Edible Native Plants of the Rocky Mtns. U. of New Mexico Press, 1967.
Harris, Ben C. Eat the Weeds, Keats Pub. New Cannan, Conneticut 1973.
_____ Make Use of Your Garden Plants. General Pub. New York. 1978.
Harris, Marjorie. Botanica North America. Harper Collins, New York, 2003.
Harrison, Nora. Flower Remedy Rhymes , self published, England, 1990.
Hart, Jeff. Montana Native Plants and Early Peoples, Montana Historical Society Press. '92
_____ The Ethnobotany of the Northern Cheyenne Indians of Montana. Journal of Ethnopharmacology 1981 4.
Hartung, Tammi. Growing 101 Herbs That Heal. Storey Books, Pownal, Vt. 2000.
Hartwell, Jonathan, Plants Used Against Cancer. Quarterman Pub. 1982
Hartzell, Jr. H. The Yew Tree A Thousand Whispers. Hulogosi, Box 1188, Eugene, OR 1991.
Harvey, C & Cochrane A. The Healing Spirit of Plants. Godsfield Press, Sterling Pr N.Y. 1999
Harvey Clare. The New Encyclopedia of Flower Remedies. Watkins Pub. London 2007.
Hatfield, Gabrielle. Encyclopedia of Folk Medicine. ABC CLIO Santa Barbara. 2004.
Haughton, Claire. Green Immigrants. Harcourt Brace Jovanovich. New York and London.
Hawksworth, Frank & Wiens, D. Dwarf Mistletoes, Ag Handbook 709, USDA, Wash, DC, '96
Health Canada, Native Foods and Nutrition. Medical Services Branch, 1995.
Heatherington, M. and Steck,W. Natural Chemicals from Northern Prairie Plants, Ag West Biotech Publishers, Saskatoon, Canada. 1997.
Heilmeyer, Marina. The Language of Flowers-Symbols & Myths. Prestel Pub. Munich 2001.
Heinerman, John. Encyclopedia of Nuts, Berries and Seeds, Parker Publishing, 1995.
_____ Encyclopedia of Healing Herbs & Spices. Parker Pub. N.Y. 1996.
Heinrich, Bernd. Winter World The Ingenuity of animal survival. HarperCollins. NY 2003.
Heinrich, Clark. Magic Mushrooms in Religion and Alchemy. Park St. Press, VT. 2002.
Heiser, Charles B. Jr. Of Plants and People. U. of Oklahoma Press, 1985.
Hellson, John C, Ethnobotany of the Blackfoot Indians No. 19, National Museums of Canada, Ottawa 1974.
Henderson, Robert K. The Neighborhood Forager. Key Porter Books, Toronto, 2000.
Hendrickson, Robert. Encycl of Word and Phrase Origins. Facts on File Inc. NewYork, 1997.
Hendry, G. Natural Food Colorants , Blackie and Son, Glasgow Scotland, 1992.
Henry, J. David. Canada's Boreal Forest. Smithsonian Institute. 2002.
Hilarion. Wildflowers, Their Occult Gifts. Marcus Books, Queensville, Ont. 1982.
Hobbs, Christopher. Usnea : The Herbal Antibiotic. Botanica Press. 1986.
_____ Medicinal Mushrooms, Botanica Press, Santa Cruz, 1995.
Hoffman, David. The Holistic Herbal. Findhorn Press, 1983.
_____ Welsh Herbal Medicine. Abercastle Publications, Dyfed, 1978.
_____ Medical Herbalism. Healing Arts Press, Rochester, VT, 2003.
Hole, Lois. Favorite Trees and Shrubs. Lone Pine Pub. Edmonton Alta. 1997.
_____ Perennial Favorites. Lone Pine Pub. 1995.
Holm, LeRoy G. World Weeds, John Wiley and Sons, 1997.
Holmes, Peter. The Energetics of Western Herbs, Vol 1 and 2, Artemis Press, 1989.
_____ Jade Remedies, Vol 1 and 2, Snow Lotus Press, Boulder 1996.
Hopman, Ellen. A Druid's Herbal, Destiny Books, Rochester, Vermont. 1995.
Howarth, D& Kahlee Keane. Wild Medicines of the Prairies Self Published, 1995.
_____ Native Medecines Self Published , 1995
Hozeski, Bruce. Hildegard's Healing Plants. Beacon Press. Boston, Mass. 2001.
Hsu, Hong-Yen. Oriental Materia Medica, Keats Publishing,Connecticut, 1986.
Huang, Kee Chang. The Pharmacolocy of Chinese Herbs. 2nd Edition, CRC Press, 1999.
Hu-Nan. A Barefoot Doctor's Manual. Running Press, Philadelphia, 1977.

Hudson, James B. Antiviral Compounds from Plants, CRC Press, Florida, 1990
Hudson, Rick. A Field Guide to Gold, Gemstone and Mineral Sites. Orca Pub, Victoria, 1999
Hurley, Judith. The Good Herb Wm. Morrow and Co. New York, 1995.
Hutchens, Alma. Indian Herbology of North America. Merco. 1969
Ingram, Cass. Supermarket Remedies. Knowledge House, Buffalo Grove, Ill. 1998.
Inkpen W & Van Eyk, R. Guide to the Common Native Trees and Shrubs of Alberta, Government of Alberta, Environmental Protection, 1995.
James & Keeler, Poisonous Plants- 3rd Int. Symposium, Iowa State U. Press, 1992.
Jason, Dan & Nancy. Some Useful Wild Plants, Talon Books, Vancouver, 1972.
Jiao Shu-De. Ten Lectures on the Use of Medicinals. Paradigm Pub. Brookline, Mass. 2003.
Johnson, Kershaw, MacKinnon & Pojar Plants of the Western Boreal Forest and Aspen Parkland, Lone Pine Press, Edmonton, Alberta 1995.
Johnson, L. Tending the Earth A Gardener's Manifesto. Penguin Books, Toronto, 2002.
Johnson, Leslie. Journal of Ethnobotany and Ethnomedicine. 2006 2:29.
_____ Health, Wholeness & the Land: Gitksan Traditional Plant Use and Healing. U of Alberta 1997.
Jones, Alison. Larousse Dictionary of World Folklore. Larousse, New York, 1995.
Jones, Pamela. Just Weed, History, Myths and Uses. Prentice Hall Press, Toronto, 1991.
Kamm, Minnie W. Old Time Herbs for Northern Gardens Little Brown & Co. 1938.
Kane, Charles W. Herbal Medicine of the American Southwest. Lincoln Town Press. 2007.
_____ Herbal Medicine: trends and traditions. Lincoln Town Press 2009.
Kapoor, L.D. CRC Handbook of Ayurvedic Medicinal Plants, CRC Press, Boca Raton, 1990.
Kari, Priscilla. Tanaina Plantlore. National Park Service, Alaska Region 1987.
Kaur, Sat Dharam. The Complete Natural Medicine Guide to Breast Cancer. Robert Rose Inc Toronto, 2003.
Kavash E, Barrie & Barr K, American Indian Healing Arts. Bantam Books, Toronto 1999.
_____ The Medicine Wheel Garden. Bantam Books, N.Y. 2002.
Kay, Margarita Artschwager. Healing with Plants in the American and Mexican West, The University of Arizona Press, Tucson. 1996
Kays, S & Nottingham S. Biology and Chemistry of Jerusalem Artichoke. CRC Press 2008.
Keane, Kahlee & Howarth,D. The Standing People. Saskatoon, Saskatchewan. 2003.
Kee Chang Huang, The Pharmacology of Chinese Herbs, 2nd Edition, CRC Press, 1999.
Kemp, Cynthia. Cactus and Company. Desert Alchemy, Tucson, Arizona, 1993.
Kenner D &Requena Y. Botanical Medicine: .Paradigm Pub. Brookline, Mass, 1996.
Kerik, Joan. Living with the Land:Use of Plants by the Native People of Alberta, Alberta Culture, Circulating Exhibits Program, National Museums of Canada Fund, 1981.
Kershaw, Linda. Edible & Medicinal Plants of the Rockies, Lone Pine, Edmonton 2000.
_____ Alberta Wayside Wildflowers. Lone Pine, Edmonton, 2003.
_____ Saskatchewan Wayside Wildflowers. Lone Pine, Edmonton, 2003.
_____ Manitoba Wayside Wildflowers. Lone Pine, Edmonton, 2003.
Kershaw, L. et al. Rare Vascular Plants of Alberta. U. of Alberta Press, Edmonton, 2001.
Kershaw, MacKinnon & Pojar. Plants of the Rocky Mountains. Lone Pine, Edmonton 1998.
Keys, John. D. Chinese Herbs, Charles E. Tuttle Co. 1976.
Kimmerer,Robin. Gathering Moss. Oregon State University Press, Corvallis, 2003.
Kindscher, Kelly. Medicnal Wild Plants of the Prairies. Univ. Press of Kansas. 1987.
King, Francis X. Rudolf Steiner and Holistic Medicine. Rider & Co. England, 1986.
Klein, Carol. Plant Personalities. Timber Press, Portland, Oregon. 2005.
Klein, Richard. The Green World. 2nd edition. Harper Collins, 1987.
Kloss, Jethro. Back to Eden. Woodbridge Press Pub.Co. Santa Barbara, Ca. 1975.
Knab, Sophie H. Polish Herbs, Flowers and Folk Medicine. Hippocrene Books, N.Y. 1999.

Knowles, Hugh. Woody Ornamentals for the Prairies. U. of Alberta , 1995.
Knudtson,P & Suzuki D. Wisdom of the Elders. Greystone Books. Vancouver BC 2006.
Kraft, K & Hobbs C. Pocket Guide to Herbal Medicine. Thieme, N.Y. 2004.
Kranich, Ernst M. Planetary Influences Upon Plants. Bio-Dynamic Lit. Wyoming RI 1984.
Krymow, V. Healing Plants of the Bible. Wild Goose Pub. Glasgow, UK 2002.
Kuhnlein, Harriet and Turner, Nancy. Traditional Plant Foods of Canadian Indigenous Peoples. Gordon and Breach Science Publishers. 1991.
Kuijt, Job. The Biology of Parasitic Flowering Plants, U. of California Press, 1969
Kunkele, U. & Lohmeyer, T. Herbs for Healthy Living. Parragon Pub. Bath UK 2007.
Lacey, Laurie. Micmac Medicines Remedies and Recollections. Nimbus Pub. Halifax, 1993.
Lahring, Heinjo. Water and Wetland Plants of the Prairie Provinces, Can Plains Research Center, U. of Regina, 2003
Lambert, Grant. Falling Leaf Essences. Healing Arts Press, Rochester Vermont, 2002.
Lamont, SM. The Fisherman Lake Slave and their environment: a story of floral and faunal resources. Master's thesis. U. of Saskatchewan, Saskatoon, 1977.
Langenheim, Jean. Medicinal Plant Resins. Timber Press Portland Oregon 2003.
Larsen,Henning. An Old Icelandic Medical Miscellany, Norske Akademi, Oslo, Norway '31
Lavabre, Marcel. Aromatherapy Workbook. Healing Arts Press, Vermont. 1990.
Lawless, Julia, The Encyclopedia of Essential Oils , Element Books, 1992.
LeClaire,N &Cardinal,G. Alberta Elders' Cree Dictionary, U of Alberta Press, 1998.
Leduc, M.A. The Explorers Guide to Boreal Forest Plants, Hwy Book Shop, Cobalt, Ont. 1997
Leighton, Anna L. Wild Plant Use by the Woods Cree (NIHITHAWAK) of East-Central Saskatchewan . Paper no. 101, National Museums of Canada, Ottawa, 1985
Lepore, Donald. The Ultimate Healing System. Woodland Books, Provo, Utah, 1988.
Le Strange, Richard, A History of Herbal Plants. Arco Pub. New York. 1977.
Leung, Albert. Chinese Herbal Remedies. Universe Books, New York, 1984.
Leung & Foster, Encyclopedia of Common Natural Ingredients, J. Wiley&Sons, N.Y. 1996.
Levey,M. The Medical Formulary or Aqrabadhin of Al-Kindi U of Wisconsin Press, 1966
Leyel, C.F. Elixirs of Life, Faber and Faber, London.1948
Li, Thomas. Medicinal Plants, Culture, Utilization & Phytopharmacology. Technomic Publishing, Lancaster, Pennsylvania, 2000.
Li, Thomas. Chinese and related North American Herbs. CRC Press, Boca Raton, 2002.
Libster, Martha. Delmar's Integrative Herb Guide for Nurses. Delmar, 2002.
Lininger et al. The Natural Pharmacy. Healthnotes, Prima Pub. Rocklin Ca, 1999.
L'Orange Darlena, Herbal Healing Secrets of the Orient. Prentice Hall, New Jersey, 1998.
Lock, Carolyn. Country Colours. Nova Scotia Museum. 1981
Lovejoy, Sharon. Sunflower Houses. Workman Pub Co. New York 2001.
Lu, Henry. Using Foods to Stay Young, Sterling Press, New York, 1996.
_____ Chinese Natural Cures. Black Dog & Leventhal Pub. New York, 1994
Luetjohann, Sylvia. The Healing Power of Black Cumin. Lotus Light, Twin Lakes, WI, 1998
Lyle, Katie Letcher. The Wild Berry Book, NorthWord Press, Minocqua, WI, 1994.
Mabey, Richard. Plantcraft. Universe Books. 1978.
MacKinnon, Pojar, Coupe. Plants of Northern British Columbia. Lone Pine Press, 1992.
Mailhebiau, Philippe. Portraits in Oils. C.W. Daniel Company, Essex, England, 1995.
Malmud, René. The Amazon Problem, trans by M. Stein, Spring Pub. Dallas TX, 1980.
Maloof, Joan. Teaching the Trees, Lessons from the Forest. U Georgia Pr, Athena GA. 2005.
Manandhar, N.P. Plants and People of Nepal. Timber Press, Portland, Oregon, 2002.
Maple, Eric. The Secret Lore of Plants and Flowers. Robert Hale Ltd. London 1980.
March, Kathryn & Andrew. The Wild Plant Companion. Meridian Hill Pub. 1986.
Marles, Robin. The Ethnobotany of the Chipewyan of Northern Saskatchewan, 1984. Thesis.

__________ et al. Aboriginal Plant Use in Canada's Northwest Boreal Forest. UBC Press, Vancouver, and Natural Resources Canada, 2000
McBride, L.R. Practical Folk Medicine of Hawaii. Petroglyph Press, Hilo,Hawaii, 1975.
McCune B. & Geiser L. Macrolichens of the Pacific Northwest. Oregon State U. Press, 1997
McFarland, Phoenix. The Complete Book of Magical Names. Llewellyn Pub. St Paul 1996
McGrath, Judy. Dyes from Lichens and Plants. Van Nostrand Rheinhold, 1977.
McGuffin, Nancy. Spectrum: dye plants of Ontario. Burr House Spinner, Richmond Hill '86
McIntyre, Anne. The Complete Woman's Herbal, Henry Holt, New York, 1995.
Mears, R & Hillman,G. Wild Food. Hodder and Stoughton
MELODY. Love is in the Earth, A Kaleidoscope of Crystals. Earth Love Pub. Col. 1995.
Mercatante, A. S. The Facts on File Encyclopedia of World Mythology. New York 1988
Merriam, C. Hart. Dawn of the World, Weird Tales of Mewan Indians. Arthur H. Clark, Cleveland, 1910
Meyer, George et al. Folk Medicine and Herbal Healing, Charles Thomas, Springfield, 1981
Meyerowitz,Steve. Sprout It! The Sprout House, Box 1100,Great Barrington, MA, 1993.
Meyers, Edward C. Basic Bush Survival, Hancock House, Surrey, B.C. 1997.
Miller, L &Murray,W. Herbal Medicinals A Clinician's Guide. Hawthorn Press, N.Y. 1998.
Miller, Sandra. Editor Echinacea- Medicinal and Aromatic Plants. CRC Press, 2004.
Mills S. & Bone,K. Principles and Practice of Phytotherapy. Churchill Livingstone, 2000.
_____ The Essential Guide to Herbal Safety. Churchill Livingstone, 2005.
Mills, Simon. Out of the Earth. Viking Penquin Books, Toronto. 1991.
Millsbaugh, Charles. American Medicinal Plants, Dover Pub. New York, 1974
Milne, Courtney. Visions of the Goddess, Penguin Studio, Toronto, 1998
Minnis & Elisens. Biodiversity and Native America. U. Oklahoma Press, 2000.
Mitchel, Jr. Wm. Plant Medicine in Practice. Churchill Livingstone, St. Louis, 2003.
Moerman, Daniel, Medicinal Plants of Native America. U of Michigan No. 19, 1986
Mohammed, G. Catnip & Kerosene Grass Candlenut Books, Sault Ste. Marie, Ont, 2002.
Montgomery, Pam. Plant Spirit Healing. Bear and Company, Rochester, VT 2008.
Moore, Michael. Los Remedios. Red Crane Books, 1990
_____ Medicinal Plants of the Desert and Canyon West. Museum of New Mexico Press 1989
_____ Medicinal Plants of the Mountain West, Museum of New Mexico Press '79
_____ Med Plants of the Mountain West. Revised, expanded. 2003
_____ Medicinal Plants of the Pacific West, Red Crane Books, 1993
More, Daphne. The Bee Book, Universe Books, New York, 1976.
Morelli, I. et al. Selected Medicinal Plants. University of Pisa. FAO 53/1
Morton, Julia. Major Medicinal Plants . Charles Thomas, Springfield, Illinois 1977
_____ Atlas of Medicinal Plants of Middle America, Bahamas to Yucatan. 1981
Moss, E.H. Flora of Alberta. University of Toronto Press. 1983
Mother, The. Flowers and their Messages. Sri Aurobindo Ashram Trust, India 1979.
Mourning Dove. Coyote Stories. Caxton Press Caldwell Idaho. 1933.
Mowrey, Daniel. The Scientific Validation of Herbal Medicine. Cormorant Books, 1986.
Mucz, Michael. Baba's Kitchen Medicines. U of Alberta Press, Edmonton, 2012.
Mulders, Evelyn. Western Herbs for Eastern Meridian & 5 Element Theory. Self publ. 2006.
Mulligan, G editor The biology of Canadian Weeds, 1-32 Pub. 1693 Ag Canada 1979
_____ 33-61 Pub. 1765 Ag Canada 1984
Murphy, Cristine Editor, Practical Home Care Medicine, Lantern Books, New York, 2001
Murray, Michael. The Pill Book Guide to Natural Medicines. Bantam Books, April, 2002.
_____ & Pizzorno, J. The condensed Encycl of Healing Foods. Pocket Books NY 2005.
Naegele, Thomas A. Edible and Medicinal Plants of the Great Lakes Region, Wilderness Adventure Books, Davisburg, Michigan. 1996.

Naiman, Ingrid. Cancer Salves, A Botanical Approach to Treatment. N. Atlantic Books, 99.
Nesse R & Williams G. Why We Get Sick. Vintage Books/Random House, New York, 1996.
Neuwinger H.D. African Traditional Medicine. Medpharm Sci. Pub. Stuttgart 2000.
_____ African Ethnobotany, Poisons and Drugs. Chapman & Hall, London 1996.
Newcombe C.F. unpub notes on Haida plants. Dept of Anthro. Am Mus Nat Hist. NY 1897
_____ unpublished papers. Prov Archives B.C. Victoria. 1898-1913.
Nicander. The Poems and Poetical Fragments. Cambridge U. Press, New York, 1953.
Norman,Howard. Northern Tales. Pantheon Books, New York, 1990.
Northcote, Rosalind. The Book of Herbs. John Lane: The Bodley Head, London, 1912.
Null, Gary. The Clinician's Handbook of Natural Healing. Kensington Books, N.Y. 1997.
Olive, Barbara. The Flower Healer. Cico Books, London and New York. 2007.
Ollsin, Don. Herbal Healing Journey-Playful Workbook. Aquiline Comm, Victoria,BC 1998.
Ootoova I. et al. Interviewing Inuit Elders, Perspectives on Traditional Health. Vol 5, Nunavut Arctic College, Box 600, Iqaluit, Nunavut X0Z 0H0.
Page, George. Inside the Animal Mind. Doubleday, New York, 1999.
Pallasdowney, Rhonda. The Complete Book of Flower Essences. New World Library, 2002.
Pappalardo, Joe. Sunflowers (the secret history). The Overlook Press. Woodstock NY 2008.
Parish, Coupé & Lloyd. Plants of S. Interior British Columbia. Lone Pine Edmonton 1996
Park, Willard Z. Ethnographic Notes on the Norhern Paiute of Western Nevada, 1933-40 compiled by Catherine Fowler, U. of Utah, Salt Lake City, 1989.
Parvati, J. Hygieia, A Woman's Herbal. Freestone Collective. 1978
Paturi, Felix Nature, Mother of Invention. Harper and Row Pub. New York. 1976.
Peirce,Andrea. Practical Guide to Natural Medicines. Stonesong Press. 1999.
Pelikan, W. Healing Plants. Mercury Press, Spring Valley NY 1997.
Pellowski, Anne. Hidden Stories in Plants. MacMillan Pub. New York. 1990.
Penoel,Daniel & Franchomme, P. L'Aromatherapie Exactement , Roger Jollois, France, 1990
Peneol, Daniel. Medecine Aromatique, Medecine Planetaire. Roger Jollois France 1991.
_____ & Peneol, Rose-Marie. Natural Home Health Care Using Essential Oils. Osmobiose Pub. 1998.
People of 'Ksan, The. Gathering What the Great Nature Provided. Douglas & McIntyre. Vancouver, B.C. 1980.
Peters, Josephine & Ortiz B. After the First Full Moon in April. Left Coast Press. Walnut Creek CA, 2010.
Pettitt,Sabina. Energy Medicine, Healing from the Kingdoms of Nature, Pacific Essences, Box 8317, Victoria, B.C. V8W 3R9 Canada, 1999
Phaneuf, Holly. Herbs Demystified. Marlowe and Company, New York. 2005
Pielou, E.C. The Naturalist's Guide to the Arctic. U. of Chicago Press. 1994.
Pieroni, A & Price L. Eating and Healing, Trad Food as Medicine. Haworth Press. N.Y. 2006.
Pfeiffer E. The Earth's Face and Human Destiny, Rodale Press, Emmaus, Pa. 1947.
Plotkin, Mark. Medicine Quest. Viking Penguin Books, New York, 2000.
Pojar, J & MacKinnon, A. Plants of Coastal British Columbia Lone Pine Edmonton 1994.
Pollock, L. With Faith and Physic: the life of a tudor gentlewoman. Collins & Brown,1993.
Polya, Gideon. Biochemical Targets of Plant Bioactive Comp. CRC Press, Boca Raton 2003
Pond, Barbara, A Sampler of Wayside Herbs, Chatham Press, Riverside, Conn.
Pressor, Arthur, Pharmacist's Guide to Medicinal Herbs, Smart Pub. Petaluma, CA,2000
Price, Len & Shirley. Understanding Hydrolats. Churchill Livingstone, Toronto, 2004.
_____ Aromatherapy for Health Professionals. Churchill Livingstone 1995.
Purvis, William. Lichens. Smithsonian Institution Press. Washington D.C. 2000
Quin, Frederick F. The Flora Homoeopathica. B. Jain Pub. New Delhi, India. 1997.
Radin, Paul. The Winnebago Tribe, Bur of Am Ethnology, Smithsonian Inst. 37th. 1923.

Rätsch, C. Plants of Love, The History of Aphrodisiacs. Ten Speed Press, Berkeley,1997.
_____ The Dictionary of Sacred & Magical Plants. ABC-CLIO St Barbara 1992.
_____ The Encyclopedia of Psychoactive Plants. Park St Press. 2005.
Reaume, Tom. 620 Wild Plants of North America. Nature Manitoba. Canadian Plains Research Center, U of Regina, U of Toronto Press. 2009.
Reckeweg, Hans-Heinrich, Materia Medica, Vol 1. Aurelia-Verlag GmbH, Baden Baden 1996.
Reich, Lee. Uncommon Fruits Worthy of Attention, Addison-Wesley Pub. 1991.
Reid, Daniel, A handbook of Chinese Healing Herbs, Shambala, Boston, 1995
Rhode, David. Native Plants of Southern Nevada. U of Utah Press. 2002.
Richards B & Kanecko A. Japanese Plants- Know Them &Use Them. Shufunotomo, Tokyo 1995
Richardson, David. The Vanishing Lichens. David and Charles, Vancouver, BC, 1975
Riddle, John M. Eve's Herbs. Harvard U Press. Cambridge Mass. 1997.
_____ Goddesses, Elixirs and Witches. Palgrave MacMillan. England 2010.
Rister, Robert. Healing Without Medication. Basic Health Pub. N. Bergen, N.J. 2003.
Roberts, Jonathan. The Origins of Fruit and Vegetables. Universe Pub. New York. 2001.
Robicsek, F. The Smoking God: Tobacco....Norman: U. of Oklahoma Press, 1978.
Robinson, Peggy. Profiles of Northwest Plants. Far West Book Service. Portland, OR 1979
Rogers, Dilwyn. Edible, Medicinal, Useful & Poisonous Wild Plants of the Northern Great Plains —South Dakota Region. Buechel Memorial Lakota Museum, St. Francis,SD, 1980.
Rogers, Pattiann. Firekeeper:New & Selected Poems. Milkweed Editions, 1994.
Rogers, Robert Dale. Sundew Moonwort Vols-1-7, self-published. Edmonton 1995-present.
_____ Rogers' Herbal Manual. Karamat Wilderness Ways, Edmonton, 2000.
_____ & Capital Health, Herbal Drug Interactions. Mediscript Comm. 2003.
_____ The Fungal Pharmacy, The Complete Guide to Medicinal Mushrooms and Lichens of North America, North Atlantic Books 2011.
Rombi, Max. Phytotherapy. Herbal Health Publishers. U.K. 1990.
Rosengarten,Jr. F. The Book of Edible Nuts. Walker and Co. New York. 1984.
Ross, Gary. Nature's Guide to Healing. Freedom Press, Topanga, Ca. 2000.
Ross, Ivan. Medicinal Plants of the World. Vol 1 Humana Press, Totowa, New Jersey. 1999.
_____ Vol 2 Humana Press, Totowa, N. J. 2002.
Rotella, Rev. Alexis. The Essence of Flowers, Jade Mountain Press, N.J. 1991.
Royer F. & Dickinson R. Plants of Alberta. Lone Pine Pub. Edmonton, AB. 2007.
Rudginsky, Marlene The Flower Speaks. U.S. Games Systems, Stamford, Conn. 1999.
Rupp, Rebecca. Red Oaks and Black Birches , Storey Comm. Garden Way Publishing. 1990
Russell, Sharman Apt. Anatomy of a Rose. Perseus Pub. Cambridge, Mass. 2001.
_____ An Obsession with Butterflies. Perseus Publishing 2003.
Ryan, J et al, Traditional Dene Medicine. Lac La Martre NWT, 1993.
Ryden, Hope. Wildflowers around the year. Clarion Books, New York. 2001.
Ryrie, Charlie. Garden Folklore That Works. Reader's Digest. Pleasantville, NY 2001.
Sagadic O. & Ozcan M. Food Control 2003 14.
Salmon, Wm. Botanologia: The English Herbal. London: I. Dawkes, 1710.
Sandberg & Corrigan. Natural Remedies, their origins and uses. Taylor & Francis 2001.
Sanders, Jack. The Secrets of Wildflowers. The Lyons Press, Guilford, CT, 2003.
Sapolsky, Robert. The Trouble with Testosterone. Scribner, New York. 1997.
Sauer, Johann Christopher, Compendious Herbal-see Weaver below.
Savage, Candace. Bees, Nature's Little Wonders. Greystone Books. Vancouver 2008.
Schalkwijk-Barendsen, Helene. Mushrooms of Western Canada . Lone Pine Pub. 1991.
Schar, Douglas. The Backyard Medicine Chest. Elliott&Clark Pub. Washington, DC. 1995.

Scheffer, Mechthild, Bach Flower Therapy, Theory and Practice, Healing Arts Press, 1988
Schenk, George. Moss Gardening. Timber Press, Portland Oregon. 1997.
Schnaubelt, Kurt. Medical Aromatherapy. Frog Ltd. Berkeley CA. 1999.
Schneider, Anny. Wild Medicinal Plants. Key Porter Books, Toronto. 2002.
Schnell, Donald. Carnivorous Plants. 2nd Ed. Timber Press, Portland, Oregon, 2002.
Schofield, Janice. Discovering Wild Plants. Alaska Northwest Books. 1989.
_____ Nettles. Keats Publishing, New Canaan, Conneticut, 1998.
Schulman, Robert. Solve It With Supplements. Rodale Press. New York. 2007.
Shapiro, R & Rapkins J. Awakening to the Plant Kingdom, Cassandra Press 1991.
Shauenberg, Paul and Paris. Guide to Medicinal Plants. Keats Publishing, 1977.
Shook, Edward Dr. Advanced Treatise on Herbology . Reprint Health Research.
Shosteck,Robert. Flowers and Plants. Quadrangle/The New York Times Book Co. 1974.
Siegfried, EV. Masters Thesis, Ethnobotany of the Northern Cree of Wabasca/Desmarais. U of Calgary, Alberta. 1994.
Silverman, Maida. A City Herbal. David R. Godine , 1990.
Silvertown, Jonathan. An Orchard Invisible. U of Chicago Press. 2009.
Simonot, Danielle. Bio-Manufacturing in Saskatchewan- Assessment of the Manufacturing Potential of Select Saskatchewan Plants, Sask. Nutraceutical Network, Saskatoon, 2000
Simpson, Brenan, M. Flowers At My Feet, Hancock House, Surrey, B.C. 1996.
Sionneau, P. An Introduction to the Use of Processed Chinese Medicinals. Blue Poppy Press, Second Printing 2003, Translated by Bob Flaws.
Smagghe, Guy Ed. Ecdysone: Structures and Functions. Springer Sci 2009.
Small, E & Catling, P. Canadian Medicinal Crops, NRC Research Press, Ottawa 1999.
Small, Ernest. Culinary Herbs, Second Ed. NRC Research Press, Ottawa, 2006.
_____ Medicinal Herbs, NRC Research Press, Ottawa, 2000.
_____ Top 100 Food Plants. NRC Press, Ottawa. 2009.
Smith, Andrew. Strangers in the Garden, the Secret Lives of Our Favorite Flowers.McClelland & Stewart 2004.
Smith, Annie Lorrain. Lichens, Cambridge at the University Press, 1921.
Smith, Harlan, Ethnobotany of the Gitksan Indians of B.C. Edited by B. Compton, B. Rigsby, and M.L. Tarpent, Mercury Series, Can Ethno Service, Paper 132, Can Mus of Civil. 1997.
Smith, Huron H. Manataka American Indian Council. www.manataka.org.
Snell, Alma Hogan. A Taste of Heritage. Crow Indian Recipes and Herbal Medicines. University of Nebraska Press 2006.
Soule, Deb. The Roots of Healing, A Woman's Book of Herbs. Citadel Press, 1995.
Spencer, Kate. The Magic of Green Buckwheat ,Richard Clay, England, 1987.
Spinella, Marcello. The Psychopharmacology of Herbal Medicine. MIT Press, 2001.
Steedman, E.V. The Ethnobotany of the Thompson Indians of British Columbia. 1930.
Stein, Sara. My Weeds, A Gardener's Botany. Harper and Row, 1988.
Stern, Gai. Australian Weeds. Harper and Row, Australia 1986
Stern Wm. Stern's Dictionary of Plant Names for Gardeners. Cassell Pub, London, 1972
Stewart, Hilary. CEDAR. Douglas & McIntyre. Vancouver/Toronto, 1984.
Storl, Wolf D. Healing Lyme Disease Naturally. NorthAtlantic Books, Berkeley, CA 2010.
Strehlow,W & Hertzka,G. Hildegard of Bingen's Medicine Bear & Co. Santa Fe 1988
Stuart, David. Dangerous Garden. Harvard University Press, Cambridge, Mass. 2004
Sturdivant L.&Blakley,T. Medicinal Herbs in the Garden, Field and Marketplace Bootstrap Guide, San Juan Naturals, Friday Harbor,WA, 1999.
Sumner, Judith. The Natural History of Medicinal Plants. Timber Press, Oregon, 2000.

Swanton, J.R. Haida Texts and Myths. Bureau Am Ethnol, Bull #29. Smithsonian Inst. Washington, D.C. 1905.
_____ Bureau of Am Ethno 26th Ann Report. Smithsonian Inst. Washington, 1908.
Szczeklik, Andrzej. Kore: On Sickness, the Sick and the Search for the Soul of Medicine. Counterpoint Berkeley 2012.
Tainter, D& Grenis A, Spices and Seasonings , VCH Pubishers, New York, 1993.
Talalaj,S.& Czechowicz,A S. Herbal Remedies, Hill of Content Press, Melbourne, 1989
Taylor, Wm &Farnsworth,N. The Vinca Alkaloids, Marcel Dekker, New York, 1973.
Teeguarden, Ron. The Ancient Wisdom of the Chinese Tonic Herbs. Warner Bros. 1998.
Telesco, Patricia. The Victorian Flower Oracle, Llewellyn Pub. St. Paul 1994
Temple, Robert. The Genius of China. Simon and Schuster. New York. 1986.
Thompson, Gerry, Astral Sex to Zen Teabags. Findhorn Press, 1994.
Thoreau, Henry David. Wild Fruits. W. W. Norton & Co. New York, 2000.
Throop, Priscilla. Hildegard von Bingen's Physica. Healing Arts Press, Vt. 1998.
Tick, Edward. The Practice of Dream Healing. Quest Books Wheaton, Illinois, 2001.
Tierra, Michael. The Way of Herbs- revised Pocket Rooks, New York, 1998.
Tigner, Daniel. Canadian Forest Tree Essences, self published,1998. ISBN 0968365809
Tilford, Gregory. Edible and Medicinal Plants of the West. Mountain Press, Missoula 1997.
Timbrook, Jan. Chumash Ethnobotany. St. Barbara Mus, Heyday Books, Berkeley Ca 2007.
Traill, E.C. Studies of Plant Life in Canada. A. S. Woodburn, Ottawa, 1885.
Traill, C. P. The Backwoods of Canada. McClelland and Stewart. Toronto. 1846.
Tobyn, G., Denham, A., Whitelegg, M. The Western Herbal Tradition. 2000 years of medicinal herbal knowledge. Churchill Livingstone Toronto 2011.
Toop, Edgar W & Williams, Sara. Perennials for the Prairies. U of A&Saskatchewan. 1991.
Treben, Maria. Health Through God's Pharmacy. Wilhelm Ennsthaler. 1982.
Tresidder, Jack. Symbols and Their Meaning. Friedman/Fairfax Pub. 2007.
Tucker A. & DeBaggio,T. The Big Book of Herbs. Interweave Press. Loveland CO. 2000.
_____ The Encylcopedia of Herbs. Timber Press, Portland. 2009.
Turkington, Carol. The Home Health Guide to Poisons and Antidotes, Facts on File 1994
Turner, Nancy J. Food Plants of Interior First Peoples. UBC Press, Vancouver, 1997.
_____ Food Plants of Coastal First Peoples. UBC Press, Vancouver, 1995.
_____ Plant Technology of First Peoples in B.C. UBC Press, Vancouver, 1998.
_____ et al. Thompson Ethnobotany. Memoir #3, Royal B.C. Museum, 1996.
_____ Plants of Haida Gwaii. Sononis Press, Winlaw, B.C. 2004.
_____ The Earth's Blanket. Douglas & McIntyre. Vancouver. 2005.
Turner, N & von Aderkas, P. Common Poisonous Plants and Mushrooms. Timber Press 2009
Turner, W.B. Fungal Metabolites, Academic Press, London and New York, 1971.
Twitchell, Paul. Herbs The Magic Healers. Eckankar, Box 3100 Menlo Park, CA, 1986.
Vermeulen, Nico. Encyclopedia of Herbs. Whitecap Books, Vancouver B.C. 1998.
Viereck, Eleanor, G. Alaska's Wilderness Medicines. Alaska Northwest Pub. 1987
Vitt, Marsh and Bovey, Mosses, Lichens, and Ferns, Lone Pine Press, 1988.
Vogel, A. Swiss Nature Doctor. A. Vogel, Switzerland. 1952
_____ Nature-Your Guide to Healthy Living. Verlag A. Vogel, Teufen, Switzerland 1986.
Vogel, Virgil. American Indian Medicine, U. of Oklahoma Press, Norman, 1970
Walker, Barbara. The Woman's Dictionary of Symbols&Sacred Objects. Csstle Books, 1988.
Walker, Marilyn. Wild Plants of Eastern Canada. Nimbus Pub. Halifax NS. 2008.
Ward, Bobby J. The Plant Hunter's Garden. Timber Press, Portland. 2004.
Ward-Harris, Joan.More Than Meets the Eye, The Life and Lore of Western Wildflowers Oxford University Press, Toronto, 1983

Watanabe & Shibuya. Pharmacological Research on Traditional Herbal Medicines. Harwood Academic Publishers, 1999.
Watt, John, and Breyer-Brandwijk, Maria The Medicinal and Poisonous Plants of Southern and Eastern Africa . E and S. Livingstone. Edinburgh and London. 1962.
Watts, Donald. Elsevier's Dictionary of Plant Lore. Elsevier. 2007.
Waugh, F.W. Iroquois Foods and Food Preparation #12 Anthropological Series, Ottawa. 1916. Reprinted by Iroqrafts, RR #2, Ohsweken, Ontario N0A 1M0, 1991.
Weaver, Wm. 100 Vegetables & Where They Came From. Workman Pub. New York, 2000.
_____ Sauer's Herbal Cures America's First Book of Botanic Healing 1762-1778, Routledge, New York, 2001.
Weed, Susan. Menopausal Years, The Wise Woman Way. Ash Tree Pub. Woodstock NY, 1992
Weigle, Marta. Spiders and Spinsters. U. of New Mexico Press, Albuquerque, 1982.
Weiner, M. The People's Herbal, A family guide. Putnam Publishing, New York, 1984.
Weiss, Rudolf. Herbal Medicine. Beaconsfield Publishers, 1988.
_____ Herbal Medicine 2nd Edition. Thieme, Stuttgart, New York, 2000.
Wells, Diana.100 Flowers and How They Got Their Names, Algonquin Books, Chapel Hill,97
Westcott, Frank. The Beaver Nature's Master Builder. Hounslow Press, Willowdale, ON '89.
Westrich, LoLo, California Herbal Remedies, Gulf Pub Co. Houston, TX, 1989.
Wetzel, Suzanne et al. Bioproducts from Canada's Forests. Springer Netherlands 2006.
WHO monographs on selected medicinal plants, vol 1, 1999; vol 2, 2002.
White, Ian. Australian Bush Flower Essences. Bantam Books, 1991
White, Florence. Flowers as Food . Jonathan Cape. 1934
Whitmont, Edward. Psyche and Substance. North Atlantic Books. 1980
Wilkinson, Kathleen. Trees and Shrubs of Alberta. Lone Pine Books, Edmonton 1990.
_____ Wildflowers of Alberta. U of A/Lone Pine Books, Edmonton 1999.
Williams, Jude. Nature's Gentle Cures. Sterling Publishing. New York. 1997.
Williamson, Darcy. 130 Medicinal Plant Monographs of the NW. self pub. E-book. 2011.
Williamson, E. Major Herbs of Ayurveda. Churchill Livingstone, Elsevier Science, 2002.
Winston, David. Herbal Therapeutics. HT Research Library Broadway NJ 8th Ed 2003.
_____ & Maimes, S. Adaptogens: Herbs for Strength, Stamina and Stress Relief. Healing Arts Press, Rochester, Vermont 2007
Wolf, Adolf Hungry, Teachings of Nature/Good Med Book,#14 Box 844 Invermere 1975.
Wolfson, Evelyn. From the Earth to Beyond the Sky. Houghton Mifflin Co. Boston, 1993.
Wood, Matthew. The Book of Herbal Wisdom. North Atlantic Books, Berkeley, 1997.
_____ Seven Herbs: Plants as Teachers, North Atlantic, Berkeley, 1986.
_____ Vitalism, the history of Herbalism, etc. N. Atlantic, Berkeley 1992.
_____ The Practice of Traditional Western Herbalism. N. Atlantic, Berkeley 2004.
_____ The Earthwise Herbal. Two vols. North Atlantic, Berkeley, 2008 and 2009.
Wood, Rebecca. The New Whole Foods Encyclopedia, Penguin Arkana, New York, 1999.
Worwood, Valerie. The Fragrant Heavens. New World Library. Novato CA, 1999.
Wren, R.C. Potter's New Cyclopaedia of Botanical Drugs and Prep. C.W. Daniel, 1988.
Wright, Clarrisa D. Food What We Eat and How We Eat . Ebury Press, London, 2000.
Wu, Jing-Nuan. An Illustrated Chinese Materia Medica. Oxford U Press. New York 2005.
Wulf-Tilford M. & G. All You Ever Wanted to Know About Herbs for Pets. BowTie Press, 1999
Yance Jr, D. Herbal Medicine, Healing and Cancer. Keats Publishing, Chicago, 1999.
Yang Shou-zhong. The Divine Farmer's Materia Medica. Blue Poppy Pr, Boulder, Co 1998.
Yang Xinrong. Encyclo Reference of Traditional Chinese Medicine. Springer Berlin 2003.
Yarnell, Eric et al. Clinical Botanical Medicine. Mary Ann Liebart Pub. NY 2002.
Yeager, S et al. New Foods for Healing. Prevention Health Books, Rodale Press, 1998.

Ying, Jianzhe, et al. Icones of Medicinal Fungi from China. Science Press, Beijing 1987
Young David et al. Cry of the Eagle, Encounters with a Cree Healer, U of Toronto Press, '89
Young, Jane & Hawley, Alex. Plants and Medicines of Sophie Thomas. 2nd Ed. 2004.
Yun, Henry. Herbal Holistic Approach to Arthritis. Dominion College. 1988.
Zevin, Igor V. A Russian Herbal. Healing Arts Press, Rochester, Vermont. 1997
Zheleznova, Irina. Northern Lights, Fairy Tales of the Peoples of the North, Progress Publishers, 1976.
Zinmeister & Mues. Bryophytes-Their Chemistry... Clarendon Press, Oxford, 1990.

FLOWER ESSENCE RESOURCES

Aditi Himalaya Flower Essences, 15,Jaybharat Society, 3rd Road, Khar (W), Bombay 400 052, India.

Alaskan Flower Essence Project, P.O. Box. 1369, Homer, Alaska USA 99603-1369. www.alaskanessences.com.

Australian Bush Flower Essences. Australia. www.ausflowers.com.au.

Bach- Healing Herbs English Flower Essences- in Canada by Self Heal Distributing, Box 95008, Whyte Postal Outlet, Edmonton, AB T6E 0E5, 1800-593-5956 or www.selfhealdistributing.com Also www.healingherbs.co.uk or www.fesflowers.com

Bailey Flower Essences, 8 Neslon Road, Ilkley, West Yorkshire England, LS298HN. www.flowervr.com

Bloesem Remedies. Netherlands. www.bloesem-remedies.com

BrynaHerb Essences. www.brynaherbessences.uk

Canadian Forest Essences, PO Box 29128,1996 W. Broadway, Vancouver, BC V6J 1Z0

Canadian Forest Tree Essences. Ottawa. www.essences.ca. 613-725-9764.

Choming Flower Essences. www.mkprojects.com

Clear Path Essences. www.clearpathessences.com

Dancing Light Orchid Essences. Fairbanks, Alaska. www.orchidessences.com

Desert Alchemy, PO Box 44189, Tucson, Arizona, USA 85733. www.desert-alchemy.com.

Deva Flower Essences BP3 38880, Autrans, France. www.lab-deva.com

Eastern Flower Herbal Essences. julied@hfx.eastlink.ca.

Falling Leaf Essences. Box 78, Kallista, Victoria 3791, Australia. www.advancedalchemy.com.au.

Findhorn Flower Essences, Morayshire, Scotland IV36 0TY. www.findhornessences.com

Florais des Minas, Rua Albita, 194-Sala 408, Cruziero, CEP 30310-160,BH, MG, BRAZIL

FlorAlive®, Brent Davis. Contact info@floralive.com

FES Flower Essence Society, PO Box 1769, Nevada City, California, USA, 95959. www.fesflowers.com

Canadian Distributor- Self Heal Distributing, Box 95008, Whyte Postal Outlet, Edmonton, AB T6E 0E5 – www.selfhealdistributing.com

Green Hope Farm Flower Essences, PO Box 125, Meriden, New Hampshire USA 03770

Green Man Tree Essences. www.greenmantrees.demon.co.uk.

Habundia Flower Essences. c/o Peter Aziz. PO Box 90, Totnes, Devon, England TQ11 0YG.

Harebell Remedies. Scotland. ellie@harebellremedies.co.uk.

Hawaiian Gaia Flower Essences. www.gaiaessences.com

High Sierra Flower Essences. PO. Box 4275 Truclee, CA 96160.

holly.hsb@highoctavehealing.com

Horus Flower Essences- horus@floweressences.de.

Hummingbird Remedies, PO Box 50161, Eugene, Oregon, USA 97405

Icelandic Flower Essences. www.kristbjorb.is.

Jade Mountain Flower Essences, Box 125, Mountain Lakes, New Jersey USA 07046-0125

Korte Phi. www.PHIessences.com

Light Heart Essences. England. www.lightheartessences.co.uk.

Light Mountain Flower Essences, Michael A. Vertolli, 1-800-667-HERB.

Living Essences of Australia, Box 355, Scarborough, 6019, Perth, Australia. www.livingessences.com.au

Living Flower Essences, www.livingfloweressences.com . Rhonda Pallasdowney.

Master's Flower Essences, 14618 Tyler Foote Rd Nevada City, California, USA, 95959.
www.masteressences.com

Miriana fortem Flower Essences. www.mirianaflowers.com and info@miraflowers.com.

naturaSacredplay, PO Box 32, Buckhorn, New Mexico, 88025, (505-535-2255).

New Millenium Flower Essences of New Zealand. info@nmessences.com.

New Zealand New Perception Flower Essences, PO Box 60-127,Titirangi, Auckland 7, NZ

Pacific Essences, Box 8317, Victoria, B.C. V8W 3R9. www.pacificessences.com.

Pegasus Products, PO Box 228, Boulder, Colorado, USA 80306-0228. 1-800- 527-6104.

Perelandra, Box 3603, Warrenton, VA. 22186. www.perelandra-ltd.com

Petite Fleur Essence, 8524 Whispering Creek Trail, Fort Worth, Texas, USA 76134.
www.aromahealthtexas.com

Prairie Deva Flower Essences, Box 95008, Whyte Postal Outlet, Edmonton, AB T6E 0E5
1-(780) 433-7882. www.selfhealdistributing.com

Ravenworks- joni@ravenworksministries.org

Running Fox Farm PO Box 381,Worthington, Maryland USA 01098

Star Peruvian Flower Essences. Santa Barbara. www.starfloweressences.com

Stars of the Meadow, David Dalton, Lindisfarne Books, Mass. 2006.

Sun Essences. Norfolk, England. www.sunessence.co.uk

Sweetwater Sanctuary Essences. www.plantspirithealing.com

Tree Frog Farm Flower Essences. www.treefrogfarm.com

Whole Energy Essences, PO Box 285, Concord, Mass. 01742

Wild Rose Essences. www.wildrose.com

Woodland Essence, PO Box 206, Cold Brook, New York, USA 13324.

11586784R00133

Made in the USA
Monee, IL
13 September 2019